# POSITIVE HEALTH

## DESIGNS FOR ACTION

W9-CGV-306

# POSITIVE HEALTH

## DESIGNS FOR ACTION

**Wesley P. Cushman, Ed. D.**
Professor, Department of Physical Education
The Ohio State University

**Mary K. Beyrer, Ph. D.**
Professor, Department of Physical Education
The Ohio State University

**Marian K. Solleder, Ph. D.**
Associate Professor, Department of Physical Education
The Ohio State University

**Robert Kaplan, Ph. D.**
Consultant in Health and Fitness
American Medical Association

CHARLES E. MERRILL BOOKS, INC.    COLUMBUS, OHIO

*Library of Congress Catalog Card Number: 65-27523*

PRINTED IN THE UNITED STATES OF AMERICA

# PREFACE

Some of the most pertinent personal health decisions facing the young adult are the focus of this book. POSITIVE HEALTH—DESIGNS FOR ACTION explores these vital problems in a highly selective manner, and through presentation of the possible choices and desirable designs for action, gives direction to the achievement of optimal health. The basic principles underlying the most effective choices and designs are also highlighted.

The eight chapters of the Preliminary Edition of this book represented the combined thinking of four individuals. Following its initial drafting, each chapter was reviewed by each of the four authors, discussed in a "conference of the four," rewritten and then reviewed again. Thus, each chapter reflected a cooperative effort.

To more fully ascertain that all the choices, designs, and problems were presented in an objective helpful manner, the 1964 edition of the text was tested in classrooms at The Ohio State University and reviewed by health educators and specialists both at The University and in various sections of the United States. These reviews were carefully read and evaluated by each of the authors and, where appropriate, changes were made. Thus, each chapter in this 1965 edition again reflects the consensus of all four authors, and, in addition, the ideas of their colleagues and health educators in many parts of the country.

We are indebted to the following people for valuable comments and suggestions on chapter content in the 1964 edition of the text: John E. Horrocks, Ph.D., Professor of Psychology, The Ohio State University; Melvin S. Rheins, Ph.D., Professor of Microbiology, The Ohio State University; Wallace Ann Wesley, Hs.D., Assistant Director, Department of Community and Health Education, American Medical Association; W. W. Bauer, M.D., Director Emeritus, Bureau of Health Education, American Medical Association; Bertram D. Dinman, M.D., D.Sc., Associate Professor of Preventive Medicine, The Ohio State University; Mrs. Rollin Brown, the National Foundation. We are also indebted to our students and our colleagues for suggestions concerning this edition.

The 1965 edition of POSITIVE HEALTH—DESIGNS FOR ACTION is presented for your use in the hope that the designs will bring choices for effective action.

> *Wesley P. Cushman*
> *Mary K. Beyrer*
> *Marian K. Solleder*
> *Robert Kaplan*

*June, 1965*

# TABLE OF CONTENTS

# CHAPTER ONE—*YOUR HEALTH—*
## *CHOICE OR CHANCE?*

Han Skal Leve! Cheers! Here's to your health! On the special occasions when these words are uttered and your friends seek to honor you, your health or well-being is often the subject of their toast. Have you ever stopped to consider *why*, when there are few things that we take more for granted than our health? As long as we have the strength and energy to do what we want to do, we go merrily along our way with little thought to our well-being, per se. To most of us, health is either "good" or "bad." However, when we pause to consider, we recognize that *health* means many things to many people.

To some people, health is primarily a matter of *chance*: "I may or may not catch a cold;" "I may or may not get poison ivy;" "I may or may not die of lung cancer, regardless of how much or how little I smoke." "It's all a matter of chance, anyway!" To other people, health is definitely a matter of *choice*: "I have a tuberculin test every year;" "I prefer to eat a good breakfast every morning;" "I make it a point to get a booster shot for tetanus routinely." Many of our routines or "health habits" are the result of choices that we once con-

1

sciously made, and that now have become automatic in our daily schedules.

Perhaps the real questions are: What are the choices, and what are their bases? What are the chances, and on what are they based? Can the right choices counteract the casualness of sheer chance? What about *you?* Is *your* state of health primarily a matter of choice or chance?

According to many textbooks, health is a specific condition, although in everyday language health may be simply "what makes you tick." Actually, a textbook definition has much to offer for our consideration. Most formal definitions of *health* imply that it (1) is a state, condition, and quality; (2) incorporates a functioning coordination of the physical, intellectual, emotional, social, and spiritual factors; (3) is a means to an end (for example, happy, satisfying living) and not an end in itself; (4) varies in degree from one individual to another and from one day to another; (5) may be described as *optimal* insofar as the ultimate in degree is concerned; and (6) is reflected in a wholesome attitude toward ourselves and society.

Definitions of health which incorporate the majority of these characteristics are:

> Health is the quality, resulting from the total functioning of the individual, that empowers him to achieve a personally satisfying and socially useful life.[1]

> Health is optimal personal fitness for full, fruitful, creative living.[2]

> Health is a state of physical, mental, and moral equilibrium, a normal functioning of body, mind, and soul. It is the state when work is a pleasure, when

[1] Edward B. Johns, Wilfred C. Sutton, and Lloyd E. Webster, *Health for Effective Living,* Third Edition (New York: McGraw-Hill Book Company, 1962), p. 5.

[2] Howard S. Hoyman, "Our Modern Concept of Health," *The Journal of School Health,* 32, No. 7 (September, 1962), p. 253.

the world looks good and beautiful, and the battle
of life seems worthwhile.[3]

These characteristics and definitions imply that health as
a *complete* state of physical, mental, and social well-being
simply does not exist. They also imply that one's well-
being exists *for* something and not simply for its own sake.
Health is something to be used; it is a quality which should
help us live as successfully and happily as possible. A third
implication is that an individual with a congenital or acquired
disorder can have optimal health as well as anyone else
because the term *optimal* in this sense means the best or most
favorable within the given set of conditions or circumstances.
Essentially, optimal health is a matter of keeping all the
relevant factors in as high a degree of performance and
balance as possible.
   Current concepts also suggest that health is a positive
and dynamic state, rather than a negative and static one. It
is optimal when it enables you to meet your responsibilities
effectively. Thus, your health is both a resource and a
responsibility. It is a resource which gives you sufficient
endurance and fitness for everyday living as well as for times
of emergency. It is a responsibility which stipulates that your
friends, your family, and your community all have a right to
expect that you will maintain the highest possible state of
well-being. The degree or hierarchy of importance which we
place upon fulfilling our basic physical and psychological
needs as well as how we attain our proposed personal goals
form a complex "health value system." The extent to which
this value system is put into *action* is reflected in the degree
to which we accept health in a positive context and as a
resource and a responsibility.
   As a nation, we seem to be accepting these concepts to
some extent. We have not been content to leave all matters
of health to chance, but rather have developed definite,
organized, public health programs to make possible an optimal

---

[3] Samuel J. Crumbine, "What Is Health?" *News Digest* (March,
1960), p. 16.

state of health to those who will accept the responsibility. Consequently, as a nation we have the greatest longevity in history. Our life span now averages 70 years, which includes approximately 67 years for men and 74 for women of the white population and 62 and 67 years respectively for non-white men and women. These data partially reflect what the differences in the socio-economic status can mean to health and the life span. Nevertheless, our current longevity is due in part to our low rates of infant and maternal mortality and our low mortality rates from communicable diseases. Today, Americans die primarily from accidents and the non-communicable diseases, chiefly, heart disease and cancer. Because we are able to control many of the communicable diseases, these diseases now appear in the *morbidity* (illness) rates rather than the *mortality* (death) rates and statistics. The great advances in medical practice, surgical procedures, and pharmaceutical skills as well as the availability of hospital care have also played major roles in helping us attain our current health status.

We could mention many more factors which have contributed to our present health status. The high standard of living in the United States has produced better housing and better nutrition as well as more effective methods of sanitation for both the individual and the community. Our voluntary and official health organizations are extensive, as is the amount of scientific health information which is made available to the public through various communications media. We would be remiss to omit mention of various negative trends such as the increases in incidence of avoidable accidents, obesity, and physical inactivity due to lack of exercise and recreation.

We can also view public health status in another framework. Let us assume that health exists in four levels: mortality, serious morbidity, minor morbidity, and positive health.[4] The lowest level, *mortality*, is that level in which few diseases and disorders can be prevented, controlled, or even survived. Fortunately in the United States, we have advanced through and beyond this level. The second level,

    [4] "Report of the Chairman of the Technical Development Board to the Governing Council 1959-1960," *American Journal of Public Health*, 51, No. 2 (February, 1961), pp. 287-94.

*serious morbidity,* represents the level in which prevention, control, and treatment of most conditions are fairly successful. Today many of our medical personnel still are functioning within this level as they search for the causes of cancer, accidents, and congenital disorders. At a third level, *minor morbidity,* the emphasis shifts to minor illnesses such as respiratory problems and digestive disorders, which cause inconvenience and economic loss. Finally, at the highest level is *positive health*—our goal of optimal well-being in a safe and pleasant environment.

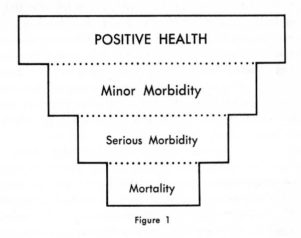

Figure 1

*Four Levels of Public Health Status*

Both the individual per se and individuals as members of a community must make intelligent choices based on the best scientific evidence and then put them into *action* if we are to attain and maintain this positive health level for acquiring optimal rather than minimal well-being. Even today, too many of us are willing to settle for as little sleep or food or exercise as is necessary to "get by." We often refuse to live to our fullest capacity! The four greatest hazards to the health of the average American citizen may well be *fear, ignorance, apathy,* and *quackery.* Perhaps the individual who is most likely to leave his well-being to chance is also most liable to fall into one of these four traps.

It is quite evident that no one person or thing can *give* you physical, mental, and social well-being to help you "to live most and to serve best."[5] Heredity already has partly determined your state of health. The physical and social pressures exerted by your environment are constantly influencing you. The values and beliefs evidenced in your home life by such specifics as eating patterns, parental discipline theories, and family recreation habits have played a role in forming your health behavior patterns. In addition you have been molded by cultural and subcultural elements including religion, race, and peer group relationships. The neighborhood in which you grew up and whether it was in a rural or urban setting in the north, south, east or west has exerted pressure.

However, much of your well-being is a do-it-yourself or problem-solving process. Its adequacy and effectiveness are dependent upon your awareness of your needs, your weaknesses, your strengths, your values, and your attitudes. Equal in importance is the knowledge that helps you determine when you can handle your health problems on your own and when you require professional help. It would be difficult, indeed, to overemphasize the part played by the specific motivating factor which prompts you to make the choice or take the chance and the role performed by your attitudes or feelings about the action in question. How easy it is for us to be motivated by attitudes and emotions, instead of facts and principles!

To expedite a successful, do-it-yourself, problem-solving program, you must base your choices and actions on scientific facts. Unfortunately, many health problems are "solved" by mere assumptions (information taken for granted without testing or knowledge of its scientific source). The ability to recognize that a problem exists, to recognize its central elements, to discard assumption, to select relevant information, and thus to make decisions based on facts and principles that have been sifted from mere opinions—such skills constitute the foundation for a scientific, not a haphazard, approach to making wise choices.

---

[5] Jesse Feiring Williams, *Personal Hygiene Applied* (Philadelphia: W. B. Saunders Co., 1950), p. 13.

A major purpose of all health instruction is to *transmit* information that the research scientist has discerned to be basic to the maintenance of health. This is step one of a two-step process. This knowledge must then be *applied* and used by both individuals and communities. This is step two. Without the application the fact is useless! Of course, it is to be acknowledged that health facts will change as the researcher discloses new information; therefore, we cannot assume that our health practices of today will necessarily be those of tomorrow. However, the current gap between what we know and what we do is appalling. We have only to consider the thousands of needless deaths from cancer each year, deaths which could have been prevented if a physician had been consulted when the first symptoms appeared. Scientists have shown us how to *decrease* dental caries, mental illness, and some types of heart disease and cancer, how to *prevent* poliomyelitis and rheumatic fever, and how to wipe out tuberculosis. Our failure to use this knowledge is costly in both dollars and lives. Health instruction attempts to reinforce the fourth level of the health status levels, the level of *positive* health. But it is up to you to initiate the action that is necessary to acquire this level—you as an individual and you as a member of a community.

One of the basic purposes in this textbook is to acquaint you with certain basic scientific principles, truths, and guidelines regarding your health and to guide you to additional authoritative sources of information so that you may apply them as designs for action to solve your health problems. Such problems may include how to handle your tensions effectively, how to approach marriage and parenthood realistically, how to begin to protect yourself now against heart disease and cancer, how to cope with environmental health problems, and how to be an intelligent health consumer. Positive, optimal health is reflected in wise choices to solve such problems. These choices, in turn, reflect the application of scientific principles that are coupled with an honest appraisal of problems and a recognition of attitudes and desires.

Positive health *is* a matter of sound, accurate *choices!* Positive health reflects a sound, effective design for action!

# Problems for Your Consideration

1. Consider some specific aspects of the "cultural lag" in our society that may be involved in our attitudes concerning the leading causes of death such as heart disease, cancer, and accidents.

2. How do apathy, quackery, fear, and ignorance retard the solution of some of our current *national* health problems? Our *personal* health problems?

3. What are some of the reasons that might explain the difference in the sex and color factors pertaining to longevity? What are the implications of these reasons?

4. Name some specific examples in which a gap may exist between what the medical researcher has discovered and what is practiced by the individual.

# Suggested References

Hein, Fred V. and Dana L. Farnsworth, *Living*. Chicago: Scott, Foresman and Company, 4th ed., 1965, Chapters I and III.

Schifferes, Justus J., *Healthier Living*. New York: John Wiley & Sons, Inc., 2nd ed., 1965, Chapter I.

United States Department of Health, Education and Welfare, *The Costly Time Lag*. Public Health Service Publication No. 813, Washington, D. C.: U. S. Government Printing Office, 1961.

———, *The Facts of Life and Death*, Public Health Service Publication No. 600 (Revised 1963). Washington, D. C.: U. S. Government Printing Office, 1963.

Williams, Jesse Feiring and Angela Kitzinger, *Health for the College Student*. New York: Harper & Row, Publishers, 1963. Chapter I.

# CHAPTER TWO—*INCREASING YOUR PSYCHOLOGICAL EFFECTIVENESS*

The college environment today encourages the fullest possible development of the individual. It is an environment which fosters a desire for learning, reflective thinking, and social responsibility. Yet, unfortunately, 40 per cent of the young people who start college do not finish. The reasons for drop outs are many and varied, but poor grades take the highest toll. Many intelligent students get poor grades because "their energies are used up trying to resolve emotional conflicts."[1]

When the student comes to college, he is given a measure of freedom that demands considerable maturity. In many instances he is just becoming independent of parental and other adult supervisors. In college he is asked to make a great many decisions for himself. He must organize his mode of life in a new environment in a way that is satisfying to himself but in a manner that is acceptable to his peers and college authorities. He must also meet certain academic requirements to be "successful."

---

[1] Dana L. Farnsworth, "Emotional Problems of College Students," *Feelings and Their Medical Significance*, 6, No. 10 (Columbus, Ohio: Ross Laboratories [November-December, 1964]), p. 1.

To be responsible for directing and controlling one's own life is no small order. It demands psychological effectiveness, that is, the ability to modify behavior to meet the demands of a changing environment. Psychological effectiveness requires certain personal skills and competencies such as the ability to understand oneself, to plan ahead, to control one's emotions, and to meet one's problems intelligently. This chapter is designed to assist you in developing a concept of personality in order that you may better understand yourself and others, to stimulate your interest for further study, that you may refine your concept in light of new and greater knowledge, and to help you to develop plans for action to improve both your personality and your psychological effectiveness.

## HOW PERSONALITY DEVELOPS

Your *personality* is the sum of your characteristics, and it develops through the learning process as you react to your environment.[2] Both biological and environmental factors shape your personality. The old argument as to which is more important, heredity or environment, is fruitless. Nature and nurture play interdependent roles. Heredity is important, but we know that most genetic dispositions can be altered by environment. For example, a boy may inherit a physique potential of six feet, two hundred pounds, but perhaps disease, an accident, or malnutrition keeps him from attaining this physique. Biological factors related to heredity affect adjustment and personality indirectly. Studies show that in junior high school the bigger and stronger youngsters hold more class offices and have greater status than their smaller and weaker peers. These large youngsters also develop different ways of adjusting in comparison with their smaller classmates, who often are smaller only because heredity determined that

---

[2] For discussion of various personality theories, see Richard S. Lazarus, *Adjustment and Personality* (New York: McGraw-Hill Book Company, 1961) and Joseph M. Wepman and Ralph W. Heine, eds., *Concepts of Personality* (Chicago: Aldine Publishing Company, 1963).

they mature physiologically more slowly than their peers. Heredity is also a factor in certain health conditions and is considered in the chapters on marriage and noncommunicable diseases.

After birth, the social environment begins to influence the child's personality. The individual is born with physiological drives and possibly, to a limited extent, with some psychological strivings.[3] These compel him to satisfy personal needs. His social environment requires that he satisfy these in acceptable ways.

All people have the same general needs, which can be roughly classified as physiological, social, and self. *Physiological needs* are hunger, thirst, sex, activity, and rest. *Social* and *self needs* include a sense of belonging, feelings of affection, feelings of being wanted, and a desire for respect and success. Throughout life the individual strives to meet these needs. How he meets them is conditioned by factors in his environment such as the values and customs of his parents and companions, the laws of the land, the taboos of society, and the teachings of his school and church. If he matures in such a way that he has self-confidence and self-control, and in so doing develops behavior patterns that are reasonably satisfactory to himself and to his society, he is well adjusted.

## DIRECTING BEHAVIOR

Basic patterns of the eventual adult personality are acquired early in life. The *unconscious* mind plays an important role in directing behavior. Authorities in personality development point out that experiences related to infant feedings, toilet training, and sex training no longer remembered by adults may be strong forces in determining how they react to certain situations. For example, the helpless baby's life centers about getting food. He cries when he is hungry. If his mother comes and feeds him, he learns that

[3] James C. Coleman, *Personality Dynamics and Effective Behavior* (Chicago: Scott, Foresman & Company, 1960), p. 114.

crying is an effective way of relieving his hunger tensions.
If he gets no response, he learns that there is no way to relieve
a painful situation. Though this example is somewhat simpli-
fied, such early experiences could lay the foundation for
developing the attitude of either trying to do something about
a problem or merely being apathetic about it.[4] Drives and
responses that are suppressed in early childhood and youth
and cannot be talked about may be unconscious throughout
life. (This may be due to the child's inability to communi-
cate or because discussion of such drives is not permitted or
encouraged by his parents.)

An infant can only demand and receive, but as he grows
and develops, he learns that he must consider others. His
parents and others discipline him by spanking, scolding, and
explaining. Thus, he gradually develops a *conscience*. Conscience is a significant part of personality and is directly
related to feelings of guilt. The girl brought up in a good
home is likely to have strong feelings of guilt if she enters
into premarital sexual relations. The teachings of her home,
school, and church have produced a conscience that tells her
such behavior is wrong. The conscience serves as a governor
and directs the mode of expression of basic urges and drives.
To avoid punishment or gain reward, the child behaves
according to the rules of those about him. At first, the
pressures to behave in certain ways are forced upon him.
They are external. As he grows and reacts he makes them part
of himself. As he begins to see himself as an individual, the
external pressures give way to become values for self-guidance
based on preference and self-respect. The mature person uses
his conscience rather than fear to direct his behavior.

*Conscious* mental activity is voluntary and can be controlled. In adjusting to his environment man can be self-
directing. He is superior to animals because of his higher
mental processes: memory, intelligence, imagination, and judgment. He can call on these mental assets in choosing a course
of action. Unfortunately, many of us never develop the skills
of planning ahead and problem solving. We muddle through

---

[4] Lazarus, *Adjustment and Personality, op. cit.,* p. 91.

without using the information the sciences have given us. We never learn how to apply the scientific method to daily living. We shall discuss designs for improving our conscious behavior in the last half of this chapter.

## Mental Mechanisms

Without defining or identifying them, we have discussed the mental mechanisms of introjection, identification, and sublimation. These mechanisms are related to our growth process. *Introjection* is the process of absorbing the attitudes and ideals of those about us. Conscience partially develops this way. Most of our values and beliefs we have automatically gained from our parents. *Identification* is a mental mechanism known to most people as "hero worship." The boy imitates his favorite athlete, the girl her favorite actress. As they develop, children unconsciously imitate their parents as well as absorb their values. Two health habits which are strongly associated with this process are smoking and drinking. Young people tend to follow the pattern of their parents in the use of tobacco and alcohol. *Sublimation* is the channeling of basic drives into socially approved ways of behavior. One learns to accept approved substitute goals for sexual or other drives that are blocked. The woman who does not marry may go into a profession such as pediatric nursing or teaching, where she can express her love in a constructive manner.

There are other mental mechanisms that we have blindly learned to use to reduce our tensions and solve our conflicts. Some of the most common of these are rationalization, projection, compensation, and conversion.[5] *Rationalization* is a process in which we justify our ideas and behavior in a way that seems plausible to ourselves; for example, the young girl who has three mid-terms coming up on Monday reasons (illogically) that she should accept an invitation to date on Saturday evening with her boy friend as the date will relax her for

---

[5] For a more detailed discussion of mental mechanisms see Lawrence F. Shaffer and Edward J. Shoben, *The Psychology of Adjustment*, Second Edition (Boston: Houghton Mifflin Company, 1956), pp. 157–86.

study on Sunday. *Projection* involves blaming our failures on others; for example, the athlete who feels his poor grade is because his professor doesn't like football players. In *compensation*, we make up for some real or imaginary inadequacy by doing well in another activity; for example, the honor student who substitutes outstanding grades for his lack of athletic ability. In *conversion*, we transfer the energy of a desire we cannot express into a physical symptom or complaint, for example, the student who comes into the college health service with complaints and symptoms of diarrhea resulting, unknown to him, from anxieties about final examinations. We use these mechanisms unconsciously to defend ourselves against anxiety, self-devaluation, and emotional hurt. To use these to some degree is normal, but overdependence on defense mechanisms is dangerous. [6]

### Adaptive Responses

One's personality is evaluated according to how he reacts to situations. One can handle problems by *flight, fight,* or *compromise.* These adaptive responses are sound methods of adjusting as long as they are used to solve problems realistically. The student who finds he cannot succeed in engineering may withdraw (flight) from that area of study to pursue another. Withdrawal, in this case, comes as a result of conscious direction. Students who dodge responsibility through illness, alcohol, or excuse-making are not responding in a healthful manner. The student who is doing poorly in a required course may use the fight reaction in a constructive manner by adopting the attitude "I can lick this one" and work harder to make a respectable grade, or he may use it in a destructive way by arguing that this requirement is absurd and the faculty doesn't know what it's doing. Early childhood experiences may very well determine whether or not the fight and flight reactions are expressed in desirable or undesirable ways.

---

[6] Coleman, *Personality Dynamics and Effective Behavior, op. cit.,* p. 205.

In compromise, one adjusts to both his own demands and those of the situation. The college sophomore gives up the idea of buying a sports car with money he earned during the summer when he realizes such an expenditure would require him to work during the school year. A job would take a great deal of his study time. He realizes that good grades throughout college may mean the difference between being placed in a highly desirable job or a less desirable one. He gives up the temporary pleasure and peer status the car would give him for a more important future goal. One learns to weigh the results, to accept what will be best in the long run.

## Mental Illness

As we noted previously, personality develops through learning, and many of our learned reactions and behavior patterns develop during early childhood and adolescence and may govern us unconsciously. If these patterns are reasonably satisfactory to both the individual and the social group to which he belongs and the individual feels good about himself, he is well adjusted. However, this is not always the case. In growing up, people sometimes develop ways of behavior that are extreme or inappropriate to the situation. If such behavior persists and interferes to the degree that one does not function effectively in his daily living, he is mentally ill. Perhaps the difference between the normal and the neurotic person is the extent of conflict with which he has to struggle. Or perhaps some people, because of their greater problem-solving ability, can better resolve their tensions. Then again, some people may be more subject to conflicts because of strong innate drives.[7]

Compared with the behavior of the mentally healthy person, the behavior of the emotionally disturbed or neurotic person is different more in degree than in kind. Anyone may become afraid of deep water under certain circumstances, but some individuals, without knowing why, have a persistent

[7] Lazarus, *Adjustment and Personality, op. cit.,* p. 94.

and excessive fear of water. One would expect to have a feeling of weakness *(asthenia)* if he were unexpectedly asked to report to the Dean. But some people have persistent and excessive weakness throughout the day for no obvious reason *(neurasthenia)*. One expects to feel elated or depressed at various times and in various situations, but a few people have periodic attacks of melancholia or elation so marked that they cannot function with any degree of effectiveness in their daily living (manic-depressive psychosis).

The mental disorders just discussed have their origin in faulty personality development and are classified as neuroses or psychoses. The neurotic person usually does not need hospital care, but his effectiveness is impaired and he does need counseling to avoid severe personality difficulties. Psychoses are more severe than neuroses and the psychotic usually requires institutional care. He withdraws, loses touch with reality, may show personality disorganization such as overexcitement and marked depression, or may have delusions of grandeur or persecution.[8] The causes of the neuroses and psychoses are not known. Development is complex and not specific. In the case of psychoses there may be inherited tendencies which lower resistance to stress.

Some mental illnesses have a physical basis. The cause can be determined. Such illnesses are termed symptomatic as the disturbance is a sign of an organic disease such as a brain tumor, tertiary syphilis, or arteriosclerosis. Mental disturbances may also be produced by an overexposure to chemicals or drugs. Many of these mental disorders with known causes can be prevented or cured by established techniques.

## DESIGNS FOR IMPROVING PSYCHOLOGICAL EFFECTIVENESS

After giving some thought to this brief discussion of how personality develops, you may have concluded that at your age there is little hope for you to change your basic per-

---

[8] Coleman, *Personality Dynamics and Effective Behavior, op. cit.,* p. 230.

sonality. You are partially correct. Even if you could appraise yourself objectively, intellectual knowledge of human development does not provide principles that you can apply to alter your unconscious patterns of behavior. However, conscious learning continues at any age. College provides you with opportunities to improve your self-image, your feelings of self-esteem. You can develop academic and social skills and competencies that will help you gain social approval. You can become knowledgeable about certain principles which, if conscientiously practiced, can improve your psychological effectiveness in handling your daily living problems. This will result in an increase in your happiness and productivity.

### Apply the Scientific Approach to Daily Living

The scientific approach, as we have mentioned before, refers to the method of gathering and examining facts and using them to reach the best possible conclusion. At the same time, one realizes that new facts may necessitate changes in decisions and plans of action.

It is not easy to apply this approach to our daily living as it requires objectivity, and in many situations the student may feel insecure or threatened and seek to protect himself. Yet, it is important for us to learn to use this approach as conflicts are part of living, and the way we handle them is important to our emotional and social life. You might begin to practice this approach by gathering facts on these questions about yourself.

*How do others see me?* Outward personality is important to success in a society such as ours that places emphasis on appearances. How would you rate yourself on agreeableness, oral expression, manners, and "looks." These are personality traits that you can consciously improve. The know-how is available. Rate yourself, then see if your friends and acquaintances agree with your ratings.

*Are my goals realistic?* Keep your goals high. Most individuals tend to underrate themselves, and some exaggerate their shortcomings to the degree that they feel inferior. Goals also can be unattainable. If, for example, you plan to be a doctor, you must be of high intelligence and able to maintain an "A" or high "B" average in college. If aptitude and psychological tests and past academic grades show little likelihood of such high performance, you may rightly conclude that your goal of becoming a physician is unrealistic. No one should decide on the result of a single test, but if a series of predictors contraindicate success in achieving a goal, you would do well to reconsider your aims. Analyzing yourself in relation to goals is difficult. If you have doubts, you should seek professional help from the appropriate counselor.

*Do I face reality?* You must learn to accept what you cannot change or control. The college girl who thinks she can change her fiancé after marriage will be disturbed when she realizes this usually cannot be done to any significant extent. The driver who kills a child through no fault of his own may develop a deep-seated emotional problem unless he carefully thinks through the situation and recognizes that such things can happen—even to him. Do you realize that fear, anger, sex drives, frustrations, stress, and guilt feelings are normal and that it is how you function with them that should be your concern?

*When do I need help with a problem?* If you have difficulty in college without understanding why, you should seek competent help from the appropriate authority or agency. Many students can avoid academic difficulties if they seek help from a college advisor rather than some classmate or fraternity brother. One needs competent help if he questions whether or not college is worthwhile, if his grades are not what they should be even though he is studying, if he is missing a lot of classes or examinations because of vague physical complaints, if he is always at odds with his instructors or people of authority, if he is depressed most of the time, and if he loses interest in others and tends to withdraw. Colleges have advisors for personal problems as well as curriculum and medical advisors. The large university may provide special marriage, legal, financial, occupational, and psychiatric counseling as well. All of us need help from time to time. Do you seek competent help when necessary?

## Face Peer Pressures Intelligently

College freshmen are always more or less pressured to adapt a pattern of behavior that identifies them with the upperclassman. Unfortunately two symbols of maturity that can quickly be copied and for which there may be readiness because of parental example are smoking and drinking. The use of tobacco and the misuse of alcohol may have serious effects on health. Smoking is often begun by girls to impress others of their worldliness and sophistication and by boys to show their manliness. The risks of smoking are discussed in Chapter Six.

The drinking of alcoholic beverages is a social custom which college students will probably encounter some time during their four years. For many it is not whether you drink but how and when you drink. Driving under the influence of alcohol has great risks and is discussed in Chapter Seven. It is interesting to note that studies show that the majority of college girls who lose their virginity during college do so under the influence of alcohol, that the majority of young men who contract the venereal diseases for the first time do so under the influence of alcohol. Although alcohol does not increase the sexual desires, it impairs the judgment.

These problems could have been discussed under our first principle, Apply the Scientific Approach to Daily Living, but since peer pressures can be great, they have been given special mention here. Get the facts; don't let the "it's the thing to do" attitude mislead you. The mature individual thinks for himself.

## Develop Intellectual Skills

To improve mental efficiency, you should know that mental work follows the same law of function as does physiological work. You know that to develop a high level of swimming ability, you must swim. The same holds for intellectual skills. If you want to learn how to write, you must write. You might get a good grade by copying a theme, but all you learn is how to copy. Learning comes through your own efforts. All the professor can do is guide your experiences.

Many students do poorly in their academic work because they have not learned how to use their time well. They do not plan a weekly study schedule. Take out your class schedule and reproduce it on a larger scale. Put your courses on in red pencil—your life must revolve around your studies. Fill in other fixed times such as employment, meals, band, and sports. What you have left must be used for study, play, and rest. Set up your day time study hours carefully. Study after your classes by revising your notes in relation to the past assignment. Work out your schedule so you know what to study when. Your schedule is only a guide, but if used wisely it can improve your efficiency and give you more time. Your schedule must be flexible enough to allow for change but when tough assignments are made, borrow your time from study hours with light assignments. Do not steal time.[9]

Inability to concentrate is the most common study complaint. Physical or psychological distractions may be to blame. Studies show that noise interferes with higher mental task output. Even music can adversely affect study which requires critical thinking, though routine thinking may not be disturbed. In any case, if your room is noisy and interruptions by others frequent, it is wise to study elsewhere. The psychological factors that serve as distractors to concentration are related to anxieties—worries about grades, the girl friend, or conditions at home. If such psychological distractions persist so that they continually interfere with effective study, the help of a counselor should be sought.[10]

Don't let low grades floor you—find out why you get them.

[9] George J. Dudycha, *Learn More With Less Effort* (New York: Harper & Row, Publishers, 1957), p. 189.

[10] William W. Farquhar, John D. Krumboltz, and C. Gilbert Wrenn, *Learning to Study* (New York: The Ronald Press Company, 1960), pp. 49-66.

## React, but React Favorably

You should not suppress your emotions but rather learn to control them. Control means utilizing an emotional drive in a wholesome rather than unwholesome manner. Control of emotions such as fear, anger, and sex can be accomplished through conscious effort.

*Fear* is a basic emotion that is common to humans. Everyone has anxieties over finances, health, family life, and his own personal adequacy from time to time. *Worry* has been described as inefficient thought whirling about a pivot of fear. Even mild anxieties definitely hamper one's ability to think clearly. Every student has experienced poor results on an examination because he was so anxious about his grade that he could not concentrate on the test. Fear also impairs memory and perception. It affects people physically. It increases the heart and pulse rate, produces a dryness in the mouth, increases perspiration, and causes one to feel chilled and weak in the knees. Stress with anxieties over a period of time is the cause or a contributing factor of certain *psychosomatic* (mind-body) diseases as ulcers, hypertension, and colitis.[11]

The best way to deal with fear is to act. If you have a problem causing you to worry, you should ask, "Is this my problem?" A lot of people worry about things outside of their control. If it is your problem, a second question might be, "Is this my problem now?" If not now, you should make a note on your calendar when action must be taken. For example, suppose you are having difficulty in composition and have a theme to turn in Friday. You might worry about it all through the week, and the anxiety would hamper your study of other subjects. Instead, you should make a note; "Write English theme Wednesday evening; rewrite Thursday a.m. 10-12." You should then do it as well as you can and forget it. There is nothing that builds self-confidence as well as being prepared.

---

[11] John E. Gibson, "Science Looks at Your Fears," *Today's Health*, 38, No. 1 (January, 1960), p. 6.

A way of dealing with fears is to identify them and develop the skills to carry on despite them. Remember that all humans have fears. If you can do nothing else, talk them out with a friend, instructor, counselor, minister, or doctor. No one is a coward because he fears.

*Anger* is a perfectly normal reaction. It has been estimated that the average man gets angry about six times a week and the average woman three times weekly. Men are more apt to get upset by inanimate objects such as a faulty car battery or some event such as tardiness. Women get angry at other people more frequently than men. The neurotic person has many pet peeves over which he gets angry. The well adjusted person usually does not get angry unless thwarted in some manner. The well adjusted person can take a kidding without getting mad; the neurotic person gets irritable.[12]

Even though anger is normal, its frequency can be reduced. Plans for action which can be helpful include recognizing hostility as a fact, identifying situations that cause anger, and developing ways of preventing it from becoming chronic. Avoid discussion of difficult problems when you are hungry or fatigued. A discussion with Dad about those low grades will go better in the early evening after a good dinner. Don't bottle up anger, but rather, talk out your difficulties with a friend or interested person. A socially accepted way of expressing daily aggressions is through physical exercise. Over a period of time, failure to express anger may produce the same psychosomatic disease as we mentioned in our discussion of fear.

*Sex* is one of our strongest drives, yet because of the taboos of our society, it often is not discussed openly. The result is that many young people misunderstand it. The sex drive or feeling becomes evident in the full sense to the young man and woman at the time of puberty. It comes on suddenly in the male and gradually in the female. Responsiveness to the drive differs between the sexes. In the male it is

---

[12] John E. Gibson, "What Makes You Mad?" *Today's Health*, 38, No. 4 (April, 1960), p. 16.

centered largely in the reproductive organs. In the female it is more diffused. In the male it is largely physical and is quickly aroused and satisfied. In the female it is more socio-psychological and is usually not as easily aroused. Men respond strongly to the biological attractiveness of the female; whereas, the responsiveness of the female is more to the social and personality appeal of the man.[13]

Because of social conditioning and biological differences, control of the sex drive becomes an individual matter. Certainly young men and women should think of what is best in the long run. There is little doubt that in our society nothing contributes more to successful living and emotional well-being than a happy marriage and family life. Nothing maintains or develops personal courage and self-confidence as does sincere love and affection. In Chapter Three we shall point out that marriage today emphasizes personal satisfaction with love as the foundation. It requires trust, mutuality, and unselfishness. Such a marriage is not built on a foundation of premarital sexual activity.

Since successful marriage and family life is a goal worth seeking, young people should make every effort to sublimate the sex drive. The student takes the most important step in control when he accepts happy marriage as his goal.[14] But, as the sex drive is strong, the student who accepts this goal should pick friends with similar ideals and should avoid situations that are overly sexually stimulating. There is always a strong feeling of satisfaction in being able to give up immediate and selfish pleasures for what is good for oneself and others in the more distant future. It is important that the student recognize his threshold of control. The highly erotic girl may need to deliberately plan her associations with the opposite sex to avoid situations in which she would lose control. Some physical intimacies between young couples are

---

[13] C. L. Anderson, *Physical and Emotional Aspects of Marriage* (St. Louis: The C. V. Mosby Co., 1953), p. 19.

[14] Henry A. Bowman, *Marriage for Moderns* (New York: McGraw-Hill Book Company, 1960), pp. 163-74.

expected, but these should not go beyond the point where the self-respect and health of either partner are threatened.

### Relieve Tensions Through Recreation and Relaxation

Daily tensions are bound to build up in our fast moving, status-seeking society. Relief can be provided through recreation and relaxation. Recreation may take many forms and provides opportunities for expressing aggressions and creativeness. You should consider two factors in selecting your own form of recreation. First, you should be able to schedule the activity frequently throughout the week. Second, you should pick out an activity that involves skills different from your work. For example, a man in a standing or sitting job who receives orders or complaints from others might be wise to select a competitive, big muscle activity in which he can express his aggressions in a wholesome manner and improve his muscle tone and circulation. The girl who practices dancing each day for a musical comedy might be wise to curl up with a good book or play a game of bridge. College provides you with many opportunities to learn leisure time activities that you can carry on throughout adult life.

Learn to relax. Too many people feel guilty about loafing. Doing nothing a few minutes each day will help you to tackle your work with enthusiasm. Some psychiatrists feel that muscle tension actually causes anxiety. It is possible with practice to learn to relax completely. Of course, adequate amounts of sleep and rest are essential in preventing tensions. Minor irritations become major conflicts to a tired person.

### Recognize That Mental Health Is a Family Responsibility

If you have understood our discussion of introjection, identification, and sublimation, you now realize that the family is the institution which plays the greatest role in shaping personality. For the most part, parents determine whether or not the child can make mistakes without being overwhelmed by them, whether or not he is game to try new things, how he feels about the world around him, and how he feels about himself.

Parents may favorably shape the personality of their child if they will stand by him when he gets in trouble, show him by their actions that they love him, let him know what is expected of him, and be consistent in their punishment of him. They should strive to follow these suggestions, which are agreed upon by most mental health authorities. Parents should answer the child's questions honestly but only to the extent that he can understand the answer. They can help him learn from his mistakes without being ashamed of them. They can assist him to become independent, to grow at his own pace, and to gain self-confidence by showing pleasure when he does well. They can teach him to be honest and sincere; studies indicate that people who have these characteristics have many fewer anxieties than those who don't have them. The young person who learns to tell the truth doesn't have to remember what he said. Parents can help him to establish worthwhile goals. Frequently youths who do not have good parental models and controls recognize this. They should consider and then follow the activities of the many wholesome adult models in society.

If conscientiously applied, the above designs for action can do much to improve your psychological effectiveness. Although by the time you are in college your basic personality is somewhat fixed, you can continue to consciously improve your self-direction. Your life must have purpose and often to achieve purpose you have to learn to pass up momentary pleasures. Some of you will make wealth your long range goal; others will choose power. But there is evidence to show that the most successful and happy people are those who have learned to satisfy their self needs through service to others.

# Problems for Your Consideration

1. What personality traits can you consciously improve through your college years? How?

2. Discuss the implications of the statement that "one must learn to function with feelings of guilt, anger, and fear."

3. Under what circumstances might stress or anxiety be constructive forces in our lives?

4. To what extent is appropriate adjustment to the sex drive a mental health problem?

5. Discuss the campus resources available to assist in the solving of student problems.

# Suggested References

Blaine, Graham B., Charles C. McArthur, and others, *Emotional Problems of the Student.* New York: Appleton-Century-Crofts, 1961.

Coleman, James C., *Personality Dynamics and Effective Behavior.* Chicago: Scott, Foresman & Company, 1960.

McKinney, Fred, *Psychology of Personal Adjustment.* New York: John Wiley & Sons, Inc., 3rd ed., 1960.

Menninger, Karl, *The Human Mind.* New York: Alfred A. Knopf, Inc., 3rd ed., 1947.

Program Area Committee on Mental Health, *Mental Disorders, A Guide to Control Methods.* New York: American Public Health Association, 1962.

Selye, Hans, M.D., *The Stress of Life.* New York: McGraw-Hill Book Company, 1956.

Strecker, Edward A., Kenneth E. Appel, and John W. Appel, *Discovering Ourselves.* New York: The Macmillan Company, 3rd ed., 1959.

# CHAPTER THREE—*PLANNING FOR*
## *A SUCCESSFUL MARRIAGE*

Whether or not to marry is, for most of us, a decision with a foregone conclusion. We expect to marry. The pressing issues are With whom? When? and What are the chances for a successful marriage?

Campus marriages are more numerous than ever before. Even high school marriages have been increasing in number. The chances for success depend, as they always have for all marriages, on a complex of factors. Pregnancies leading to marriage, illegitimate births, early age at marriage, and school dropouts are problems which are reflected in our high divorce rates.[1] There is no simple answer to how you can assure yourself of success. We shall discuss mate selection and marriage through some of the issues and characteristics which can contribute to its success. The choices are yours!

---

[1] Hugh Carter and Alexander Plateris, "Trends in Divorce and Family Disruption," *Health, Education, and Welfare Indicators* (September, 1963), pp. v-xiv, and Helen E. Martz, "Illegitimacy and Dependency," *op. cit.*, pp. xv-xxix.

## WHY WE MARRY

Though you may not realize it, "old-fashioned" reasons
for marriage are not extinct. Your great-grandparents were
probably influenced strongly in their younger days by the
prevailing social reasons for marriage. To a lesser extent,
these same reasons affected your parents' marriage. Many
marriages today are made for the same reasons.

Not long ago it was considered practical for a man to
marry in order to have children who could help with agricultural and housekeeping tasks. This is still true in parts of
the world where children are needed, for example, for hunting
and fighting. Among the wealthy, children—particularly males
—are a means of maintaining the family name, protecting
accumulated riches, and even establishing a measure of
immortality. Among the nobility, even today, arranged
marriages are a means of enhancing political and economic
fortunes.

The woman's need for security in the predominantly
"man's world" of years ago was of greater importance than
today. She had to depend upon the family structure for both
social and economic security. Today she can be socially and
economically independent. For this reason, it is possible
for a woman to remain single, pursue a career, and live a
satisfying and happy life. Many women elect a career and
are quite successful, too.

Housekeeping and childbearing have always been important contributions, even though women did not always receive
the recognition they deserved for these abilities. However,
when they were limited to only these potentials, in most
instances, women either married or suffered in ignominy as
the family's "old maid." Fortunately, in today's world we
value the woman not only for the traditional reasons but also
for the variety of other roles she is capable of fulfilling.

In a more agricultural society, the husband and wife
understood the necessity for division of labor. Interdepend-
ence in the accomplishment of daily tasks for mutual benefit
and productivity was a major consideration. The man farmed,

hunted, and made tools, while the woman prepared food, kept house, sewed, and raised children. Division of labor may have been the main motivation for marriages which were arranged or contracted. Under these conditions the man also tended to meet his need for security.

Unlike the perplexing "chicken or the egg" question, it is possible to say which came first, the changes in the reasons for marriage or the changes in the roles and responsibilities of men and women. Industrialization and urbanization of society brought a variety of changes in family structure, functions, and responsibilities. During the periods of major wars, social change was accelerated and the nature of change may have been altered as well. Where members of a family of the past lived their lifetimes in one community among relatives and neighbors who knew them well, today's average family moves once almost every five years.[2] Where grandparents and even aunts and uncles used to live in one household, today's family unit includes only mother, father, and children. Sociologists call the former the *extended family* and the latter the *nuclear family*. The individual is no longer as strongly dependent upon the family. Where children's friends and boy-girl relations were very closely supervised by family and community, today their freedom to choose friends and move about unsupervised is almost unlimited.

At the same time that family ties loosened, the economic reasons for marriage changed. Needs for children, security, and division of labor are no longer necessary reasons for marrying. Most of the needed services such as food preparation, laundering and cleaning, clothes making, and tool making are readily available. Only the satisfactions of intimate sexual relations are more difficult to procure in our society—and even their availability is subject to question. If we have less need to marry, and families no longer give as much social, economic, and psychological support to our marriages, why then do we marry?

---

[2] United States Bureau of Census statistics show that 20 per cent of the population moves each year. Assuming that different families move every year, within five years time all will have moved once. See also, Ruth S. Cavan, *The American Family* (New York: Thomas Y. Crowell Company, 1953), p. 72.

## Love

Perhaps some individuals are still motivated to marry for traditional reasons. To some extent, the "old" reasons are still influential in most modern marriages. The great difference between then and now is in the changed *emphasis* on the reasons for being married. Today, there is little emphasis on the necessity of joint labor for survival. Love, respect, and companionship receive more stress. The modern relationship seems to be a desirable and satisfactory means of fulfilling many psychological-personality needs. Reasons for marriage today include desires for love and affection, the security of being wanted and needed, socially acceptable means for sexual satisfaction, children, and, generally, happiness.

Thus, marriage is more satisfying and, at the same time, more difficult to maintain. There is greater opportunity for happiness, but there is also greater opportunity for poor choice and personality conflict. Reduced support from the family is a paradox, too. We enjoy freedom of choice and our own responsibility, but we miss the support and guidance that older members of the family could provide. Where marriages are arranged by elders, love, affection, and respect can develop after the wedding. This was frequently the case in grand-father's day, and it still occurs in India and other nations. Nevertheless, it can be said that we marry because of our need to love and be loved.

It is an oversimplification to say that people "marry for *love*." Books have been written on the meaning of love. Society has imposed the institution of marriage to fulfill love. However, few of us can define it. Some consider love to be an irrational force for irrational behavior. The normal developmental progression for individuals is from self-love, to parental love, to filial love, to love of those of the same sex (homosexual), and then to the love of those of the opposite sex (heterosexual). If we were to define love as an emotional attachment to some object or person, we would imply that love is unidirectional and irrational. Mature love is *reciprocal*. The feeling of "we" and "you" rather than "I" and "me" exists in both partners. Mature love is also *rational*. Over time, couples learn to accept their mates as they really are, recognize their assets and liabilities, and adjust to or accommodate differences in personality and behavior.

### Love and Premarital Behavior

Love is not *lust*. It is sexual and it may start with physical attraction, but it is not sex alone. Relationships based only on sex seldom last. The unfortunate paradox is that the sex drive is frequently the strongest at a time when marriage must be postponed. This is especially true for the man. Thus, he may seek relationships in which thoughts of sex or actual sexual behavior are emphasized.

For the woman, *cultural pressure* to have a boyfriend and to marry increases with the passage of time, or at least until she reaches an age when she is accepted as a "bachelor-girl." Too frequently, these pressures impel the girl to submit to sexual relations with the boy on the assumption that he will love her enough to marry her. Too often, the ruse fails.[3]

Whether or not to engage in premarital sexual intercourse, whether or not it will strengthen personal bonds, whether or not it is harmless, satisfying, or beneficial can be difficult choices. The problem is further compounded by the "double standard." Historically, this unwritten law or belief which still prevails considers premarital, and sometimes extramarital, sexual relations to be the prerogative of the male. In many cultures, even today, his masculinity is supposedly established by his "conquests." On the other hand, in our society a woman is expected to follow the course of chastity and fidelity. If detected in an illicit relationship, she is condemned and considered to be promiscuous. In any case, the social penalties for women in these circumstances are usually much more severe than for men.[4]

---

[3] For a more extensive discussion, see: Grace Naismith, "When the Sap Begins to Flow," *Today's Health*, 43 (February, 1965), pp. 44-46+.

[4] Joan Beck, "The Other Face of the Problem: The Unmarried Teen Father," *Today's Health*, 43 (February, 1965), pp. 28-31+.

For example, consider the laws against adultery and prostitution. Though the former is rarely enforced, in the latter, the customer (male) goes unpunished, while the seller (female) is sent to jail. Is it only because these laws were made by men? By inference, then, a woman who submits to such a relationship runs the risk of being degraded, even if only subconsciously, by the very man who seemed to find her desirable. Frequently, he does not consider such relationships as a prelude to marriage.

Sexual equality—equal sexual rights for men and women —does not prevail in our society. In spite of publicity to the contrary and effectively written appeals, sexual equality is still a long way off.[5] Whether, in the future, we become more restrictive for the male or more permissive for the female is a problem for conjecture.

Our system of values does not include premarital sexual experience as "good" for the individual or society. Even disregarding the possibilities and consequences of pregnancy, venereal diseases, loss of self-respect and mutual respect, and feelings of guilt where partners are concerned, love and marriage still depend to a considerable extent on family and community approval and support. The disadvantages of furtive "back seat" sexual relations include the inhibition of true sexual satisfaction, a misguided idea of the role of sex in marriage, and a misconception of love.

Sometimes the assumption is that since the couple is already enough in love to marry, why not have sexual relations? To answer, we first need to ask, "How much love is enough?" The standards are vague to say the least. A reasonable answer is difficult to formulate. Some of us have "been in love" several times. And several times, we may have felt this was really it! Others have never "really been in love." What course will they follow when they "fall" in love? Unfortunately, many who marry young and in haste are motivated by their glands. They later divorce in the remorseful glare of reason. At any rate, it is reasonable to suggest

---

[5] For a more extensive discussion, see: Simone de Beauvoir, *The Second Sex* (New York: Bantam Books, 1962).

that premarital sexual intercourse be evaluated in light of the almost-universal goal of happy marriage which students set for themselves. When this is done, such questions as the following arise: Is premarital intercourse a contribution to the achievement of this goal? Or is it neutral? Or is it an impediment? As preparation for marriage, is it necessary or unnecessary?[6]

This is not to imply that sexual adjustments are an unimportant aspect of love and marriage. We shall discuss this further in the next chapter.

Either by chance or by choice, most marriages succeed. Mostly *by choice,* many couples lead happily married lives. What are some of the identifiable characteristics or factors that contribute to the probability of attaining that state which we call a happy marriage?

## FACTORS IN A HAPPY MARRIAGE

### Age and Maturity

As we implied earlier, time plays a role in reducing emotional, self-oriented behavior by allowing thought and perspective to guide decisions. Normally, we develop from the selfish-immature to the more selfless-mature person. While *age* does not guarantee maturity and wisdom, the development of these qualities and the subsequent thoughtful, rational making of choices and decisions is generally associated with age. Unfortunately, many young adults reject this principle and rationalize their emotionally based thinking by labeling adult thinking as old-fashioned.

It has been said that any mature couple can make a successful, if not completely happy, marriage. (For our purposes, a marriage is *successful* if it does not terminate in separation or divorce. While there are degrees of happiness, a marriage is a *happy* one when the partners feel that it is.)

---

[6] Henry A. Bowman, *Marriage for Moderns* (New York: McGraw-Hill Book Company, 1960), p. 163.

The high divorce rates among early marriages—those of couples under twenty years of age—are evidence of the need for maturity. Women who marry in their mid-teens are considered to be three times as likely to divorce as those who marry after twenty years of age.[7] Allowing time to grow into love rather than following the popular misconception of "love at first sight" is one sign of a mature relationship. There are exceptions, of course, as in those who mature early, or those whose marriages fortunately survive stormy periods while the partners mature to a level allowing for adjustment and successful marriage. How much maturity is necessary for successful interpersonal relationships and marriage we are not able to say. Maturity is probably one thing we can't have too much of, and the more the better.

The *mature* person, in general, has a fair estimate of his own assets and liabilities; he can forego immediate satisfactions and work toward a long term goal; he can accept situations and persons without idealizing them or attempting to change them when change is not possible; he is reasonably independent; he can accept compromise and work cooperatively; and he can love someone besides himself. Mature individuals *behave* as the customs, laws, and morals of their society expect. A mature person also realizes that he may occasionally feel regret about his marital choice—"What would it be like if I had married the other girl?"—or he may even have thoughts involving infidelity. Such thoughts are normal and should not cause guilt feelings to develop. An extension of the concept of maturity includes the development of emotional stability as we implied in the chapter on psychological effectiveness.

A considerable *age difference* between marriage partners may be a problem. When the woman is considerably older, such as fifteen or twenty years, social problems may be

[7] United States Bureau of Census statistics show a divorce rate of approximately 12.6 for teen-age marriages. This is three times the 4.8 per thousand for the 21-25 year-old age group. See also, Henry M. Graham, "Teen-Age Marriages," *Journal of the Indiana State Medical Association* (August, 1962), pp. 1194-1202.

greatest. More frequently, we find husbands who are considerably older than their wives; the most obvious disadvantage is the possibility of the wife's early widowhood. Of course, a fifteen-year difference in the declining years is not as significant as in young adulthood. With male longevity increasing, the problem is being somewhat reduced. Nevertheless, the most common and most successful practice is the marriage in which the man is slightly older than his wife. In any case, it seems best to marry someone relatively close to you in age.

For college students, the likelihood of meeting and marrying one's agemate is great. Today, most couples marry when the man is slightly less than twenty-three years of age and the woman approximately twenty years. While many are older than these average ages when they marry, many are also younger. Those who marry immediately following high school graduation, or even earlier, may be giving up advantages gained by those who marry later, during or after their college years.

### Health

"If you're going to fall in love, choose someone who is rich." Paraphrasing this common expression we can say, "Choose someone who is *healthy*." Usually the subtle states of health of apparently robust young adults are not a consideration during dating and courtship. Since we will discuss premarital examinations in the next chapter, we will only indicate here the need for considering health in the early stages of courtship. A premarital examination is not likely before a couple is engaged but should be completed before the wedding date is set.

Awareness of our own health status and confidence in our hereditary background is to be expected. But what of our potential or intended spouse? Admittedly, there is difficulty in acquiring an accurate assessment of someone else's health, but isn't it wise to consider serious involvement with one whose health and heredity will supplement and complement your own? Noncommunicable illnesses such as heart conditions, diabetes, epilepsy, asthma, allergy, and rheumatism do not necessarily disqualify individuals as adequate, even superior, marriage partners. However, in addition to hereditary characteristics which might affect the children of a marriage, one should consider his own willingness and ability to carry the possible burden of medical care, special attention, and special treatment of a chronically ill spouse. Of course, when illness develops after marriage, or a handicapped child is born, we have already developed a relationship in which our feelings, attitudes, and sense of responsibility leave little room for conflict. Out of love and duty, we meet our obligations to our loved ones. Even so, such circumstances can be difficult and trying. Would we be wise to seek a relationship which starts with a handicap?

There are few absolute rules to guide us regarding *heredity*. Certainly, if no children are desired, a marriage can be made in which inheritable defects are of no concern. On the other hand, where children are desired, inherited tendencies to develop certain diseases such as diabetes, epilepsy, some forms of cardiovascular or heart and blood vessel diseases, and some forms of schizophrenia or mental illness can be important considerations. This is particularly true if a history of inherited tendencies or defects exists in the families of both partners. Inherited characteristics may be of no real consequence, but consultation with a doctor is warranted in any case. He can reduce worry and anxiety and help to avoid the destructive tendency to "fix the blame" due to misunderstanding. Some defects are congenital, due to development before birth, or are a result of birth injury. If a dominant inherited characteristic such as Huntington's chorea, a disease associated with degeneration of the brain in adults, is present, marriage is not recommended.[8]

In any event, if inheritable defects or chronic illness exist and you choose to go on and be married, you must prepare yourself to expend greater effort to experience success.

---

[8] Amram Scheinfeld, *The New You and Heredity* (Philadelphia: J. B. Lippincott and Co., 1950), p. 578.

## Personality and Courtship

*Personality* is a difficult concept to verbalize, but it is a generally understood term. The variations are infinite and the persons we like as friends or associates may not necessarily have the personalities that we could live with in a marriage partner. As we stated in the second chapter, personality is the sum of one's characteristics. It is the result of heredity and environment and is not easily changed. Choosing to spend a lifetime with a personality that is not complementary or compatible with your own would be a most grievous error. Hasty marriages with too short a period of courtship as well as early marriages whose partners have an immature realization of the nature and responsibilities of marriage, frequently run head on into personality conflicts. During dating and courtship, we tend to behave in our "Sunday best." Afterward, we are most likely to be ourselves. How then can you determine whether your potential mate wants to be the "take charge," dominant type or the "let George do it," submissive type? The saying that "like marries like" may properly be applied to interests and values, but personalities should be complementary and not so alike as to be conflicting. Time is needed to learn to know each other's personality.

In addition to the selection of partners with complementary personalities, we can recommend another principle: Happy marriage is associated with people who have enjoyed a combination of happy parents, happiness in childhood, strong parental attachments (but not too strong to break), and frank attitudes toward sex.[9]

The *courtship* and *engagement* periods allow for the most realistic appraisal of compatibility in many areas in addition to personality. The optimum length of each period depends upon the length of acquaintance, experience with the opposite sex, and knowledge of and acquaintance with each other's families. Thus, the engagement period might be relatively

---

[9] Judson T. Landis and Mary G. Landis, *Building a Successful Marriage,* (Englewood Cliffs, New Jersey: Prentice-Hall, Inc., Fourth Edition, 1963), pp. 111-112.

short—let us say, three months—if the courtship period was relatively long—let us say, one year. Both might be even shorter if the couple and their families had an acquaintance or affiliation of long standing. Evidence shows that the longer courtships—two years or so—offer the greatest chance for successful marriages. *Honesty,* a personality trait of value, is important here for at least two reasons. During courtship, it may be required to break off and avoid a marriage which, in all fairness, should not take place. During marriage, it helps to maintain the necessary element of trust.

### Interests, Goals, and Values

Interests, goals, and values are interdependent. Considered separately, common *interests* are important elements of successful, happy marriage. Most individual and mutual interests should have been identified by the time of the engagement period. Planning for making adjustments and compromises related to interests, goals, and values should continue throughout married life. To be happy, couples need not golf, garden, and go to the opera together. However, while allowing for individual interests which may be engaged in separately, there should be an ample number of mutual interests which both can pursue simultaneously.

Since *goals* are an inherent part of other factors in marital success, we need say little about them. However, mutual agreement on what a couple expects of marriage, where they want to "go" socially, how high they want to go economically, how they want to get there, what roles they will play in civic activities and community welfare, and how many children they hope to have are all goals dependent upon *values* which need consideration.

That which is valuable to one may be of no value to the other. Unfortunately, this may be a source of conflict. To collect art originals or reproductions, real antiques or imitations appear to be examples of differences only in material values. But these may be a reflection of a broader value system and sense of what is important in life. If you value good taste, good manners, and well-bred children, you should choose a partner accordingly. With increasing leisure time, affluence, and longevity, couples should consider how they will spend their future years. What they will do about the size of the family may be related to what they will do after the children are grown. What plans will they make in regard to illness or death? How will they take care of grandmother? Such questions are best answered with forethought and by couples who have similar values. Frequently, similar educational backgrounds lead to similar values and interests.

### Educational Background

Partners of equal or nearly equal *education* are more likely to have common interests and similar modes of communicating with each other. It can be a disadvantage for a high school graduate or a freshman college coed to leave school and go to work to put her husband through college and professional training. Not only are there marital hardships in the process, but too frequently the couple find they lose intellectual contact, have fewer common interests, and have fewer mutual friends after four or more years. While there are extreme differences in educational levels which can obviously lead to difficulties, marrying while in college can also lead to this type of problem. As we have implied before, there are no absolute rules and the interaction of many factors must be considered. Thus, if personalities are complementary, interests and goals are similar, and age and maturity levels are compatible, then educational differences may be overcome. Happily, most marriages where the wife "puts hubby through" do succeed and these early years are thought of most fondly. Certainly, the educational gap is not so great between wives who graduate from college and their husbands who graduate from professional schools. Another factor to be considered here is the matter of the wife's career. Some women, particularly those who are highly educated, are not completely satis-

fied by fulfilling only the roles of wife and mother.[10] They may
have the interest and the talent to pursue a career as well.
Their marriages might have included plans to pursue their
fields of interest or professions. Many women who do so
have raised families, made their husbands happy and proud,
and have made significant contributions in their work. At the
very least, they feel their educations were not wasted.

Partners will not match perfectly in all respects, but they
will have to work at reducing friction in those areas where
differences exist. Generally, the fewer differences between
backgrounds the greater the likelihood of happy marriage.

### Economic and Social Backgrounds

The similarities and compatibilities of *economic* and *social*
backgrounds are intertwined with educational background,
interests, values, and goals. Some college marriages later have
unanticipated difficulty because everything seemed to be
"even" or compatible in the campus environment. Coeds dress
alike, boys dress alike, activities are similar for both groups,
and most couples spend about the same amount of money for
dates. For both men and women, tuition, books, and living
expenses are about the same. But when the glamour of the
honeymoon wears off, a wife accustomed to the niceties
provided by her well-established father may find adjustment
to a new austerity more difficult to take. Of course, she
should consider the future earning capacity of her husband
and perhaps she should elect to work until children come.
A realistic review of the cost of living and a budget when
planning marriage can be quite sobering and helpful.

A woman who "needs" a Cadillac convertible and an
upstairs maid should not marry a chainstore grocery clerk—
unless his father owns the corporation. A man accustomed
to having servants in his home ought not consider marrying

---

[10] For a more extensive discussion, see: Betty Friedan, *The Feminine
Mystique* (New York: W. W. Norton & Co., Inc., 1963); see also, John
Lear, "Will Science Change Marriage?" *Saturday Review*, 47 (December
5, 1964), pp. 75-77.

someone from the "other side of the tracks." This may seem like a snobbish attitude, but motion pictures, which have glamorized that sort of relationship, have probably distorted our ideas of its true frequency of success. For some men, it may be still more difficult to marry a woman who is a great deal wealthier. Certainly, our democracy enables us to grow and improve our status, but where there are wide differences in backgrounds, adjustments are much more difficult and probability favors a less happy, if not unsuccessful, relationship. The greater success of marriages between college graduates may be due to a reduction of differences as well as better communication and problem solving between partners.

*Occupation* can be related to social as well as economic conflict. For example, physicians frequently have demands upon their time which interfere with home life. Some wives will want to consider carefully their husbands' occupations if they involve evenings away from home, night work, travel—or even being home too much because the office is in the home. In such circumstances, social contacts and companionship may be difficult to maintain. In the early blush of matrimony, this appears to be no problem, but over a period of time irritation may grow.

### Religious Background

When individuals marry, *religion* may not appear to be important. As with other factors, there are exceptions, but we can identify some general principles regarding the consideration of religious differences. To many couples, a church wedding is of great significance. Moreover, more successful marriages are associated with church weddings than with non-church (civil) weddings. A church wedding can be an indication that a couple take their marriage vows seriously, have the approval and support of their families and friends, and have spent time and thought in planning. When children come into a family where the parents are of different faiths, the question of which religion shall be practiced frequently causes great difficulty. When a couple are planning their wedding, it may not seem to matter much and they may make a choice readily. Later, however, religion and religious training often become more important to parents and the issue can be most difficult to resolve. Frequently, religious pressures from the relatives of both parents are very disruptive and add to the conflict—more so when grandchildren enter the picture.

*Interfaith* marriages are less uncommon with the increased mobility in our society. However, for every such marriage that succeeds, there are many that fail. Sometimes one partner adopts the faith of the other, and this may help, providing there is compatibility in other areas. Too frequently, a conflict over money, friends, or any number of other differences degenerates to include dissension over racial or religious differences. Even where man and wife are of the same race and faith, if one is conscientious about religion and the other is indifferent, a source of irritation and conflict can be present. Fortunately, for many couples religion is a unifying force that supports happy marriage.

A word about *interracial* and *international* marriage. In a campus atmosphere, interpersonal relations with many individuals of different races and backgrounds are possible, even desirable. However, with greater personal freedom and little or no social pressure against it, a marriage between individuals of different races may develop. This is ill-advised. Unfortunately, our society is not prepared to accept interracial marriage. The individuals involved are usually rejected by both races. Frequently, leaving one's homeland to live in a foreign country is disillusioning if not devastating to the individual and the marriage, particularly if race is also a factor.

### Family Approval and Support

An indication whether sensible choices are being made is the reaction of the couple's *families*. Though they are not infallible, parents and older members of the family are more experienced and have the best intentions for their children. *Relatives*, and *friends* too, frequently are more objective than the courting couple, and their reactions and feelings can be an indication of both successful choice and future support.

Though today's families are nuclear and less dependent upon their relatives, various aspects of family life are still important. Family support at weddings, births, confirmations, graduations, and deaths is generally desired. Frequently, relatives help each other during illnesses, child care, and economic crises. To discount the importance of the family is to be shortsighted indeed.

## THE COLLEGE MARRIAGE

We have already implied the advantages of longer courtship. Time is needed for the young couple's love to grow and mature, for evaluation of family relationships, and for serious consideration of the many areas in which adjustments will have to be made. At home, a more normal and realistic setting may provide an aid to a more stable and profound courtship.

Away at college, couples do not usually enjoy the guidance of their families and friends. It may be more difficult to realistically assess compatibility. Controls on behavior and environmental pressures to sober the emotions are reduced considerably. Fortunately, evidence shows that marriage among college graduates is usually more successful than among those of lesser education. However, marriage while in college may be another matter. Many such marriages fail.

There are considerations unique to the college situation: Can the couple afford to be married? Who will support them? Will they both complete their educations? If one must drop out of school, which one? If a baby comes, can they afford it? Will their situation be fair to the baby? Can they both continue to study even with a baby? Can they maintain an adequate standard of living? Can they adequately complete preparations for their desired careers? Will they grow apart if one progresses academically and the other does not?

More and more college couples are marrying and doing

it successfully. However, many say that if they had it to do over, they would wait. The difficulties of marital adjustment, loss of "college-life" satisfactions, and difficulties in completing their educations gave them cause to reconsider. What would they have lost had they waited? What could they have gained?

Considering everything, we can conclude that maintaining a happy marriage is an enviable endeavor. Where the partners have laid the proper foundation through consideration of all the areas in which adjustments have to be made and in which compatibilities already exist, the couple has the best of all possible beginnings. But the two partners do not merely "live happily ever after."

Marriage is a *two-way working* relationship. If emotional maturity is needed for choosing a partner, much more of it is needed for keeping one—particularly when a marriage starts off under trying conditions. During courtship and engagement, both partners consciously and unconsciously gather information on which to base an estimate of their mutuality of interests, affectional responses, sex attitudes, and family development. After the wedding, both partners will learn that their estimates were not entirely correct. To the extent that they are mature enough, they will make satisfactory adjustments.

Fortunately, most marriages survive. They are not only successful, they are happy. The college student has the best opportunity to make a successful and happy marriage through development and use of the ability to balance emotion with reason. As rational people, couples can search out, identify, and, *by choice,* apply those principles or factors important to their marriage. Age, personality, education, religion, and family are but a few of the factors they must consider. Within each of these are principles—rules of conduct or "laws"—which if followed can usually lead to successful marriage relationships. Since these are not absolute, we shall mention one final principle. The greater the amount of agreement on a given factor or application of a principle, and the greater the number of factors and principles agreed upon, the greater the chances of a successful, happy marriage.

# Problems for Your Consideration

1. What are the advantages and disadvantages of making a choice of a marriage partner on the basis of campus contacts only?
2. What are the special adjustments that must be made if college marriages are to be successful? What are the advantages of marriage while in college? Disadvantages?
3. Of what value is the engagement period?
4. What are some of the personal and community problems and responsibilities created by increased sexual freedom?
5. Of what significance is an understanding of the concepts of mental health when planning for marriage?
6. What types of immature behavior are likely to be detrimental to successful marriage?
7. How can you determine before marriage whether a particular person will be "easy to live with"?

# Suggested References

Calderone, Mary S., M.D., "A Doctor Talks to Vassar College Freshmen About Love and Sex," *Western Journal of Surgery, Obstetrics, and Gynecology.* 72 (March-April, 1964).

Cavan, Ruth Shonle, *Marriage and Family in the Modern World.* New York: Thomas Y. Crowell Co., 1965.

Duvall, Sylvanus, *Before You Marry.* New York: Association Press, 1960.

Gordon, Albert I, *Intermarriage: Interfaith, Interracial, Interethnic.* Boston: Beacon Press, 1964.

"Love and Marriage," *Today's Health* (special issue). 42, No. 4 (April, 1964).

Lowrie, Samuel H., "Early Marriage: Premarital Pregnancy and Associated Factors," *Journal of Marriage and Family Living.* 27:48-56, February, 1965.

Peterson, James A., *Education for Marriage.* Second Edition. New York: Charles Scribner's Sons, 1964.

"Premarital Sex Behavior: A Symposium," *Marriage and Family Living.* 24:254-278, August, 1962.

# CHAPTER FOUR—*LOOKING FORWARD TO PARENTHOOD*

With the emphasis on love and companionship in modern marriage, the role of sex becomes a more important, though not all-encompassing, factor in its success. In courtship, management of the sex drive is a major concern. Couples should realize that the drive exists normally and that it can be adequately satisfied in the proposed marriage. An important process in deciding when and whom to marry is evaluating your own and your partner's attitudes towards sex and children. Mutual agreement on forms of social behavior, interpersonal relationships, displays of affection, discussions of sex, and desire for parenthood all serve to indicate probable compatibility. A couple who have agreed to marry should have considered and begun to develop mutual concepts of the role of sex and the desirability of parenthood. In this chapter, we shall concern ourselves briefly with these subjects and a bit more extensively with an understanding of the process of human reproduction, indicating where *choice* rather than chance can have its effect.

## SEX AND LOVE

In our society, children generally represent the fruition of that profound relationship called *love*. Wives want to bear and raise children born of their love. Husbands want to father and be responsible for their wife's children. These are not children born of necessity—children required for economic or survival reasons—but the products of desire or choice. An intimate personal display of affection and respect are represented in the wholesome sexual relationship of love in marriage. Sensual satisfaction is important, but it is not the only reason for the sex act. The immature individual, the exploiter, and the domineering male of the past, who demanded sexual submission of his wife as part of her "duty," have no place in modern marriage. Present knowledge of contraception and family planning enables married couples to express and enjoy their love in its deepest sense without fear of overburdening their families or "overpopulating the earth."

Many young couples do not realize beforehand that mutually satisfactory sexual adjustment in marriage frequently takes longer to attain than other areas of adjustment. This is not true for all couples, but unrealistic expectations of sex can make adjustment difficult. Mass media such as movies, magazines, television, and advertising misinform by giving the impression that mutual sexual satisfaction is easily attained. Perhaps on more primitive levels of expression, this would be true. However, even as an act of mutual love, some of the factors that can aggravate the complexity of making a good sexual adjustment are the man's relatively quick readiness for sex and the woman's slower developing readiness, and other factors such as fatigue, poor health, fear of unwanted pregnancy, and unsatisfactory premarital experience. *Chastity* before marriage, sometimes belittled, is still a widely held value. It is also considered an important foundation for the structure of our society. Violations of moral and religious codes frequently lead to guilt feelings and conflict which can adversely affect sexual adjustment. More enlightened attitudes toward the wholesomeness of the human body, the role of sex and the sex act, and the marital relationship have made the mutual satisfaction contributing to a happy marriage possible to ever-increasing numbers of people. To the extent that we have been properly oriented toward sex and its meaning by parents, church, and education, we can more readily achieve sexual adjustment in marriage.

## THE PREMARITAL EXAMINATION

A significant aid to the reduction of problems and the attainment of adjustment in marriage is the *premarital examination*. In most states, the only requirement by law is a blood test of both partners before a marriage license is issued. If syphilis is found, the license is withheld until adequate treatment is obtained and further tests prove negative.[1] Too often, young couples believe that the blood test is an adequate premarital examination. One blood test does not constitute an examination. Many factors enter into a health appraisal.

At least several weeks—preferably a few months—before marriage the couple should be examined by a physician. Either or both partners may have had no medical checkup for several years, and to start a marriage with undetected and uncorrected defects or in poor general health would be a serious handicap. Diseases such as heart disease and diabetes which may contraindicate childbearing may be discovered. Rarely, but significantly, anatomic defects which may prohibit or affect childbearing and sexual adjustment are found. In such cases, correction and counsel by a physician is indicated. Intimate counseling with both partners on matters of sexual adjustment, fertility, hereditary characteristics, and state marriage laws may be necessary. Blood typing, particularly with reference to the Rh factor, may be considered at the time of an examination.

Making such decisions as can properly and mutually be arrived at before the wedding reduces the possibility of later difficulties. In the event that the rhythm method of contraception is to be practiced, the woman will want to see her family physician or gynecologist a few months before the wedding so that her menstrual cycle can be determined. Couples should remember that excitement such as preparation for the wedding and honeymoon may alter the cycle. Those who prefer may be given information concerning contraceptive

---

[1] Sylvester W. Trythall, M.D., "The Premarital Law," *Journal of the American Medical Association*, 187 (March 21, 1964), pp. 900-03.

pills or be fitted with contraceptive devices. For some women, the *hymen*, a membrane which partially blocks the opening of the vagina, may have to be stretched prior to sexual intercourse. Formerly, it was believed that an intact hymen was evidence of virginity. However, this membrane can be ruptured inadvertently in the course of normal activities.[2]

Too frequently, only the woman obtains premarital examinations and counseling services. The man normally has no superior education or background in these matters. He will do well to recognize his responsibilities. Though it may be preferable to visit his own family doctor for his personal examination, both partners should be present when being counseled on marital adjustment.

Not all physicians are adept at premarital counseling. Nor can they always anticipate your greatest concerns. You should be prepared to speak frankly and to ask the questions you want answered. Such matters as establishing a desirable frequency for sexual intercourse, expectations for orgasm or complete satisfaction (particularly for the woman), and sexual techniques are best discussed with the physician by both partners. Sexual adjustment in marriage can be one of the more difficult problems. For the most part, ignorance and misunderstanding contribute to it.

Clergymen, family life educators, and marriage counselors can be valuable in supplementing the counseling aspects of the premarital examination and discussions with parents. For some marriages, the value of recognizing the need for and obtaining the qualified, objective services of a counselor *during* marriage, as well as before, cannot be overestimated.

## THE PHYSICAL ASPECTS OF SEX

The sex organs of the male and female complement each other and are in some respects similar. They develop from the

---

[2] Grace Naismith, "The Premarital Examination: Its Importance to Both the Man and the Woman," *Today's Health*, 42 (April, 1964), pp. 50-51+.

same cell of the embryo, but differentiate in accord with
hereditary determinants. For example, the *prostate gland* of
the male and the *uterus* of the female originate from the same
embryonic source. The *penis* and the *clitoris* are both nerve
centers. The *testicles* of the male correspond to the *ovaries*
of the female. Beginning at *puberty*, male sex cells, *sperm* or
*spermatozoa*, are produced by the testicles, as are the hormones
which cause the development of male characteristics such as
muscular hardness, deep voice, beard and body hair. At
puberty in the female, the ovaries produce the female sex
cells, *eggs* or *ova*, and the hormones which cause the development of female characteristics such as broader hips and a more
curvaceous figure, breasts, softer skin and muscle, and a
slightly different distribution of body hair. It may be said
that a girl becomes a woman when the *estrogenic* hormones
begin to function.

### The Female

In the female, after the onset of puberty, the sex organs
undergo a continuous cycle in preparation for bearing a child.
This *menstrual cycle* is the only human function in which a
loss of blood is a sign of health rather than illness. For most
women, problems of the menstrual cycle are non-existent or
so mild as to require no alteration in normal activity. For
some, such difficulties as *dysmenorrhea*, painful menstruation,
or *amenorrhea*, absence or stoppage of menstruation, may
require medical attention to attain relief. Under the control
of the endocrine system, each month—or an approximation
thereof—one ovary produces an ovum which travels through
the *Fallopian tube* toward the *uterus. Ovulation*, or the release
of the ovum, usually occurs in alternate ovaries. Sometimes,
perhaps simultaneously, more than one egg is produced.
This can lead to the birth of fraternal twins. While the ovum
is developing, the uterus is building up a lining of blood and
lymph with which to nourish the potential *embryo* when it
arrives. If the ovum has not been fertilized by a male sperm,
it disintegrates and the blood and lymph are discharged

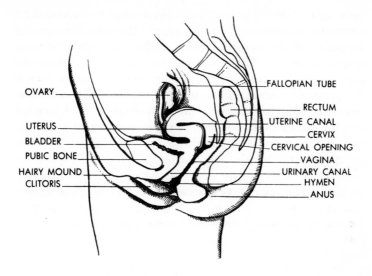

OVARY

UTERUS

BLADDER

PUBIC BONE

HAIRY MOUND

CLITORIS

FALLOPIAN TUBE

RECTUM

UTERINE CANAL

CERVIX

CERVICAL OPENING

VAGINA

URINARY CANAL

HYMEN

ANUS

**Figure 2**

*Cross Section of the Female Organs* *

* Adapted with publisher's permission from Bernard R. Greenblat, M.D., *A Doctor's Marital Guide for Patients.* Chicago 60625: Budlong Press Co., 1959.

through the *vagina* as the *menstrual flow*. The period of discharge is known as *menstruation*. The approximate periods of the menstrual cycle are: first to the fifth day, menstruation; fourteenth day, ovulation; twenty-eighth day, end of the cycle and again the onset of menstruation. Since the ovum can be fertilized for only a brief period (estimates vary from anytime up to a few hours after ovulation to two days), the fertile period occurs approximately at the middle of the cycle. However, the only certainty about menstrual cycles is their *uncertainty*. The term "approximate" is to be emphasized because of the wide variations between individual women in the schedule of their cycles and of variations within an individual from time to time.

*Menarche* is the term designating the onset of a girl's first menstruation. The age range varies widely from 9 to 16 years or so, but the average falls between 11 to 13 years old. Approximately thirty to forty years later, the ovaries will reduce the production of estrogens and ovulation and menstruation will cease. This is known as *menopause*. Though she can no longer have children, sexual relations can continue.[3] Recent developments in hormone therapy enable *endocrinologists* to consider prescribing treatment which delays or decelerates the degeneration of female organs and characteristics.

### The Male

The male sex organs are outside of the abdominal cavity and thus are more easily visualized. Their function is comparatively simpler than that of the female. There is no

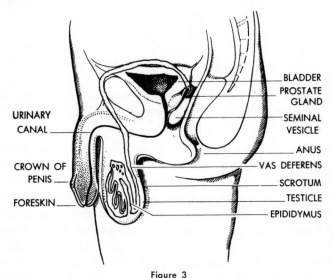

Figure 3

*Cross Section of the Male Genital Organs* *

* Adapted with publisher's permission from Bernard R. Greenblat, M.D., *A Doctor's Marital Guide for Patients.* Chicago: Budlong Press Co., 1959.

[3] For a more complete discussion, see: G. Lombard Kelly, M.D., *A Doctor Discusses Menopause* (Chicago: Budlong Press Co., 1959).

counterpart to the female menstrual cycle, and after the onset of puberty the male is, in general, continually ready to perform his role in reproduction. The testicles or *testes* are contained outside of the body in a sac called the *scrotum,* where they maintain a temperature one or two degrees lower than body temperature. Sperm are continually being produced—by the millions—in the canals of the testes and stored in a larger tube called the *epididymis.* When stored sperm become too numerous, they are released or *ejaculated* through the *vas deferens* and the urinary canal or *urethra.* The *seminal vesicle* and *prostate gland* add fluid to form *semen.* So-called "wet dreams" or *nocturnal emissions* are those quite normal occasions during sleep when excitement occurs and the male unconsciously releases accumulated sperm. Self-stimulation of the genitals, or *masturbation,* is not necessary for the release of stored sperm. Masturbation, which is normally engaged in by men more than by women, does no physical harm. However, traditional attitudes have categorized it as morally wrong. Thus, those who practice masturbation sometimes experience feelings of guilt and psychological conflict which may adversely affect their sexual adjustment. The modern point of view is less negative in its attitude toward masturbation.

### Human Reproduction

During sexual excitement the spongy tissues of the penis become engorged with blood, causing the organ to become rigid and hardened. The *erection* enables the penis, during intercourse or *coitus,* to enter the vagina so that the semen and its motile sperm (approximately 250 million of them) can be deposited by ejaculation in the vagina near the opening of the cervix—the lower portion of the uterus.

Sperm deposited in the vagina swim up into the uterus and on into the Fallopian tubes if favorable conditions exist. Movement is accomplished by the whip-like action of the tails of the tadpole-shaped sperm. *Fertilization* occurs if an ovum or egg, moving along the tube toward the uterus, meets a sperm which can penetrate its outer wall. The ovum travels

primarily by the wave-like action of the *cilia* or hairs lining
the walls of the tubes.

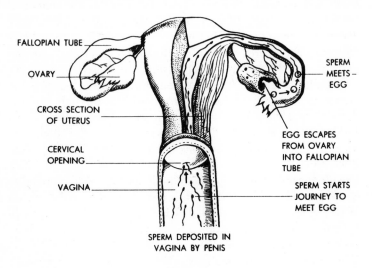

Figure 4

*The Process of Fertilization**

\* With publisher's permission from Bernard R. Greenblat, M.D.,
*A Doctor's Marital Guide for Patients.* Chicago: Budlong Press Co., 1959.

With the union of the sperm and the egg begins a process
of cell division and the potential development of a new
individual. At the time of conception hereditary traits are
determined. As cell division within the ovum takes place, the
uterus, which has been preparing itself for supporting an
embryo by storing blood and lymph, accepts the *implantation*
of the fertilized egg and *pregnancy* follows.

## PREGNANCY AND CHILDBIRTH

Among the early signs of pregnancy or *gestation* are
unusual irritability, cessation of menstruation, sensitive breasts,
and nausea or morning sickness. Frequently, the pregnancy

is well under way before some signs are observed. Since the cessation of menstruation may not be due to pregnancy, laboratory tests which identify certain hormonal changes are the most reliable indicators of pregnancy in the early stages. For example, a sample of urine is taken and injected into a test animal such as a frog or rabbit. If certain hormones are present in the urine, changes in the animal's ovaries occur indicating the probability of pregnancy. Tests are being refined which chemically analyze the urine in a few hours and which promise high accuracy in early identification of pregnancy. Occasionally such tests have to be repeated.

The embryo grows rapidly and begins to develop a placental attachment to the uterine wall. Later in the pregnancy, the *placenta* and *umbilical cord* pass food from the mother to the fetus and return wastes. After three months, the embryo is called a *fetus* and this is its designation until birth. The uterus stretches to accommodate the rapidly growing fetus, causing some displacement of other organs. The external physical changes are more visible but are only temporary. In addition to cessation of menstruation and ovulation due to hormonal action, other chemical changes occur such as the preparation of the breasts for *lactation*.

### Prenatal Care

During the pregnancy, which lasts approximately 270 days, the mother should receive adequate prenatal care from her physician or *obstetrician*. She would do well to follow sound health practices including a wholesome diet, with vitamin supplements if prescribed by her doctor. Actually, her health practices in earlier years may be more important. After the determination of pregnancy and an examination by the physician, routine visits will be made every three to four weeks for the first seven months or so. Then visits will be made more frequently—every week or two—depending upon the physician and the course of the pregnancy.

The physician usually checks to see that proper weight and blood pressure are maintained. Periodically, he will analyze the blood and urine. He may recommend that the mother give up cigarette smoking, since evidence indicates that mothers who smoke tend to have premature babies. He will check on the position and size of the fetus and measure the pelvis to determine if a cesarean section delivery is indicated. He will also check the blood for the Rh factor. (These conditions are explained later in this chapter.) In addition, during this time, arrangements for fees and periodic or prepayment plans can be worked out to reduce financial burdens.

Under proper care, various complications formerly common in pregnancies are now usually well-controlled.[4] For example, toxemia, a form of blood poisoning due to metabolic disturbances in the mother, usually occurs in women unattended during pregnancy. A mother might have heart disease or diabetes, which would require close medical supervision during pregnancy. The likelihood of premature babies, that is, those under five and one-half pounds at birth, and infant mortalities is reduced by prenatal care. While our infant mortality rate is low, prematurity is a major cause of infant deaths and is associated with various defects. (Other conditions which require medical attention are discussed later in the section on congenital defects.)

### The Birth Process

The amazing growth and complex development which lead from a minute cell, invisible to the naked eye, to a normal size baby, approximately six to eight pounds in weight and eighteen to twenty-two inches in length, is a feat of nature even more miraculous than man's harnessing of atomic power.

The process of *childbirth* is also a phenomenon of infinite magnitude. At the end of full term, and sometimes earlier, a hormonal change triggers the muscular uterine wall to start contractions. Known as *labor*, the discomforting and somewhat painful contractions are more easily tolerated with proper

---

[4] William G. Birch, M.D., *A Doctor Discusses Pregnancy* (Chicago: Budlong Press Company, 1963). (Available only through a physician.)

prenatal care and exercise and a wholesome attitude toward childbirth. Some anesthetic may be used to reduce discomfort.

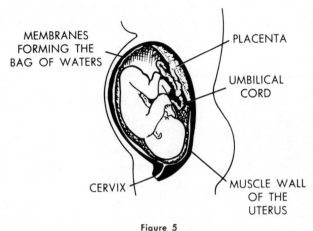

Figure 5

*Full Term Baby in Uterus**

* With publisher's permission from William G. Birch, M.D. and Dona Z. Meilach, Ph.D., *A Doctor Discusses Pregnancy.* Chicago: Budlong Press Co., 1963.

Early indications that the *first stage* of labor is about to begin are the rupture of the "bag of waters"—which is the *amniotic sac* containing the fluid which protects the fetus—perhaps a discharge of mucus, and intermittent contractions. With the fetus normally in a head-down position at this stage, contractions at the upper end of the uterus start moving the baby toward the remarkably elastic vagina, the birth canal. When the cervix is sufficiently dilated to allow passage of the head of the fetus into the birth canal, the *second stage* of labor begins. This is the actual *birth* of the baby. This stage is complete when the baby has been expelled by the force of the uterine and abdominal contractions of the mother, frequently assisted by the physician. As soon as the baby is born, mucus is cleared from its respiratory tract, the umbilical cord is cut, and silver nitrate or penicillin eye drops are used to prevent gonorrheal blindness. The *third* and *final stage* of childbirth occurs within about a half hour when the placenta and amniotic sac are expelled from the uterus. This is called the "afterbirth." The normal and natural process of childbirth which has taken place for untold generations is now safer than at any other time in history.

### Breech and Cesarean Births

Normally, babies pass through the birth canal and greet the outside world in a headfirst position. In about 3 per cent of all births, babies present themselves buttocks and feet first. These are called *breech* births. The possibility of early respiratory function during the birth process, among other reasons, increases the risk in breech position deliveries. However, when anticipated, and with special handling by the physician, most of these births are successful and cause no greater discomfort than normal births.

In some instances, the pelvic structure of the mother is too narrow, the fetus is too large, or the mother's health is such that a *cesarean section* is required. In this case, the baby is delivered through an incision made in the abdominal and uterine walls. The fetus is taken before it enters the birth canal. Women may have several cesarean sections with no difficulty. Though the dictum "Once a cesarean always a cesarean" is usually followed, a physician may, under certain conditions recommend that a subsequent pregnancy terminate in a normal, vaginal delivery.

### HEREDITY

Parents are often concerned about the hereditary characteristics which may be passed on to their progeny and the possibility of defects or mental retardation. The science of *genetics* is still comparatively young, though much is already

known about the transmission of inheritable traits from generation to generation. Genetic counseling at the time of the
premarital examination can be most helpful, particularly if
the family keeps accurate health records and medical histories.

Recent research into the structure of chromosomes and
the role of *DNA* (deoxyribonucleic acid) in the transfer of
genetic material is helping us to understand the process of
heredity.

Inheritable traits are carried by the *chromosomes* in the
*nucleus* of each cell of our bodies. Within each of forty-six
chromosomes are the multitude of *genes* responsible for
specific characteristics. In the sperm and the ovum, only half
this number of chromosomes is present. Thus, when the
two unite in fertilization, the normal number of twenty-three
*pairs* of chromosomes is restored. The element of chance
comes into play when a random assignment of chromosomes
occurs during the development of the sperm and ova. (In the
female, development of ova begins before birth and the
eggs are stored in the ovaries; in the male, sperm development occurs after puberty.) Chance continues to have its
effect in determining which sperm with its particular genetic
"message" will unite with which ovum and its particular
genetic potential.

The sex of a child is determined by chance. The male
produces two types of sex determining chromosomes, called
X and Y. The female produces only an X type. Thus, an
ovum can carry only an X sex chromosome while a sperm may
carry either an X or a Y sex chromosome. If a sperm containing a Y chromosome fertilizes the X-carrying ovum, a boy is
conceived. The boy then carries an XY pair of sex chromosomes. A female carries only the pair XX. Of course, chance
would be somewhat reduced if for some reason the male
produced one type of sperm cell which was "healthier" than
the other or the ovum tended to "select" one type of sperm
cell over the other.

Multiple births, usually twins, may or may not be hereditary. It is suspected that some women inherit a tendency
to produce more than one ovum at a time. Thus, it is possible

to have dissimilar or *fraternal* twins. A fertilized egg which splits into two separate units as the initial cell division takes place produces *identical* twins—each receiving exactly the same genetic material. In addition to a genetic tendency in the mother, the father's genes also stimulate the development of identical twins.

A principle that lends some predictability to the chances of inheriting certain characteristics comes from the *Mendelian laws* of inheritance: Genes that are paired differ in their effects. One usually dominates the other and is called *dominant;* the other gene is called *recessive.* Thus, if each parent carries a gene for the dominant trait dark eyes and a recessive gene for light eyes, the chances are one in four that the two recessive genes will combine to produce a light-eyed child. A general rule, which supports the belief that first cousins should investigate their background thoroughly before marrying, is that hereditary defects are generally *recessive* while normal traits tend to be dominant. Thus, if there is a history of a specific defect in the families of both partners, the likelihood of transmitting it to offspring is greater. A predisposition to the mental disease *schizophrenia* is probably inherited through paired recessive genes. Of course, other factors must be operative before predispositions or tendencies become manifest. A predisposition to diabetes is also considered to be inherited through recessive genes. Knowing that diabetes exists in the family should alert one to take steps to avoid its development, if possible, or detect it early so that it might be better controlled. In addition to rare inheritable cancers, a tendency to acquire cancer may be inherited. In the previous chapter we cited the inheritable disease, Huntington's chorea, which is due to a single dominant gene as are some abnormalities of the hands and feet.

## Congenital Defects

Your chances of being the parent of normal children, as opposed to abnormal children, are far greater. Estimates indicate that a little over 7 per cent of the children born have

birth defects. Of these, 3 per cent have congenital malformations which are more easily recognized at birth.[5] Actually,
almost all of us have defects to some degree.

*Congenital defects,* or birth defects, are imperfections
present at birth due to abnormal embryonic development.
Some defects, however, such as those involving the skeletal
structure, teeth, heart, and other internal organs may not be
detected at birth and do not become apparent until later life.
Many birth defects are correctable, especially if detected early.

Heredity, genetic disorders or mutations, infection, radiation illness, injury, malnutrition or abnormal nutrition, and
drugs or toxic chemicals are among the known causes of birth
defects. Since congenital means existing at and usually before
birth, defects due to injury during the birth process may
be included.

Frequently, combinations of hereditary and environmental
factors are multiple causes of birth defects. Diabetes, schizophrenia, and cancer, mentioned earlier as inheritable, are
examples of birth defects which usually appear later in life.
An inherited disposition to one of these diseases influenced by
certain environmental conditions may precipitate the disease.
An example which has received attention far out of proportion to its importance and unduly worries parents is the
"Rh disease".

The *Rh factor* is an inherited component of human blood
which was discovered in the blood of the Rhesus monkey.
Under certain conditions, this chemical factor can cause a
disabling and fatal blood disease in the human newborn. This
hemolytic disease known as *erythroblastosis fetalis* occurs in
only a small percentage of births. The problem is similar to
that which occurs when ABO blood types are mismatched
in transfusions.

When the Rh factor is present in the blood, as it is in
more than 85 per cent of the population, a person is said to
be *Rh positive.* In about 13 per cent of all marriages, the
wife is Rh negative and the husband is Rh positive. Only in

---

[5] Morris Fishbein, M.D., Editor, *Birth Defects* (Philadelphia: J. B.
Lippincott and Co., 1963), p. v.

this small group is there a possibility of encountering any difficulty and even then it can usually be corrected.

Several conditions must prevail in order to cause a "yellow baby"—jaundiced and anemic as a result of erythroblastosis. First, the unborn child must inherit the positive blood factor from its father. If the father is heterozygous—inheriting both factors from his parents—the baby may inherit his negative factor. Frequently, it inherits the mother's negative condition. Second, there must be a "leak" in the blood vessels of the placenta which allows the Rh positive blood of the fetus to mix with the mother's negative blood. Frequently, no leak occurs or is too small to be of immediate significance. Then, the mother's blood system must a) react to the presence of the Rh positive factor, b) produce antibodies with which to fight the "foreign" Rh positive cells, c) produce antibodies in dangerously large quantities, and d) pass the antibodies through the placental membrane into the blood of the fetus.

In Rh-incompatible couples, less than 10 per cent of all births are affected. Sensitivity and production of antibodies increase in mothers only if, in subsequent pregnancies, the fetus inherits the father's positive factor. Even if this allergy-like reaction (which is also similar to the development of immunity to infectious disease) develops, it is possible for the physician to control the disease.

A precautionary measure during prenatal care is to conduct periodic blood tests for the presence of antibodies in the mother's blood. Fortunately, this would occur late in the pregnancy. If severe enough, and it rarely is, the obstetrician may elect to induce early birth to remove the fetus from the now hostile environment. Also, he will be preparing to transfuse the blood of the newborn with compatible Rh-negative blood. The baby will produce Rh-positive blood which will restore itself in the system. A technique for transfusing blood when necessary into the unborn fetus is currently under development. In many ways, the Rh problem is more the concern of the physician than the parents.

While mental retardation, as well as other defects, can be caused by erythroblastosis, other diseases are more significant. *Mongolism*, for example, is the most common cause of mental retardation. This is due to a genetic disorder in which there is an extra chromosome or a translocated—misplaced—chromosome.

Infectious diseases are also a factor in birth defects. If the mother has the German measles (Rubella) during the first three months of pregnancy, there is a 20-30 per cent possibility of having a baby with a brain, hearing, vision, or heart defect. Syphilis can be transmitted from mother to fetus and defects result. Gonorrhea can cause blindness if, during the birth, the infectious organism in the vagina gets into the fetus' eyes and if appropriate eyedrops are not given.

The fact that many of these conditions are preventable or can be corrected demands greater attention. While the list of defects appears long, we must remember that most babies are born normal. In addition, there are many choices which can be made to reduce the chances of encountering serious congenital defects.

## ADDITIONAL CONSIDERATIONS

The essentials of reproduction are components of the healthy reproductive systems of the male and female: an ovum capable of being fertilized, active sperm capable of fertilizing an ovum, an unobstructed route for their passage, and a uterus favorably disposed to maintaining a developing embryo.

### Miscarriage and Abortion

A nonliving embryo or fetus that becomes detached from the uterus prematurely and is expelled is said to have *miscarried*. Miscarriage or *spontaneous abortion*, if it occurs, usually takes place quite early in the pregnancy. Studies of miscarried embryos and fetuses have shown that a vast majority were defective or abnormal. Thus, a miscarriage may reasonably be considered a blessing in disguise. Chronic miscarriage may be related to the health status of the potential mother and requires medical attention.

*Artificial* or *induced abortion* is the elimination of the embryo by chemical or mechanical means. Chemicals and drugs are not too effective and are frequently injurious, even fatal, to the mother. Mechanically induced abortion—that is, with the use of instruments—requires competent medical procedures. Under certain conditions, to save the mother, legal abortions are conducted in hospitals. Other than this, abortion is usually illegal and considered immoral. Many abortions are unwarranted—a missed menstrual period is not necessarily a sign of pregnancy. However, in increasing numbers, women with unwanted pregnancies seek unqualified "friends" and quacks to induce abortion. Consequently, in addition to great financial cost, the result is often sterility and even death due to hemorrhage and infection from injury.

### Sterility and Infertility

Either temporarily or permanently, in one or both partners, one or more of the essential components may not be met.[6] The terms *sterility* and *infertility* are used to designate this condition, though sterility is generally used to indicate a permanent condition.

Infertility can frequently be reversed. Blocked tubes, a malpositioned uterus, hormonal deficiency, inadequate quantity or quality of sperm, undescended testicles, and unfavorable emotional conditions are among the causes of infertility that are often correctable. These conditions are no reflection on one's masculinity or femininity. They may be inherited or acquired defects—perhaps due to measles, venereal diseases, or other diseases. Certainly, if children are desired, premarital examinations and postmarital counseling can be important aids to reducing infertility. However, if necessary, adoption can become a highly satisfactory alternative.

---

[6] Milton S. Godfried, M.D., "Procedure in Infertility," *Infertility and Adoption* (New York: Planned Parenthood Federation of America, March, 1953, Pamphlet material).

## Child Spacing

Children can be blessings when wanted; when unwanted, they are felt to be burdens and may suffer from rejection. To permit a newly married couple to make adequate marital adjustments, the first pregnancy should be deferred for a year, possibly two. For health reasons it is preferable for mothers to have children no less than eighteen months or two years apart. Financial as well as health considerations help to determine child spacing and the number of children a family should have. Individual couples' choices will vary widely, however.

Family planning or *birth control* is still a controversial subject. While the Roman Catholic Church opposes mechanical and chemical methods of contraception, it does not oppose the more natural rhythm method. In any case, the method of family planning—whether by pill, device, or natural methods —is a matter of individual choice. Contrary to popular belief, such organizations as the Planned Parenthood Federation have not been primarily interested in preventing births. Their main interest has always been to help families plan their growth. Currently, permissive legislation is being passed, where needed, in many locales to allow health and welfare departments to give birth control assistance to disadvantaged families who request it.[7] Thus, with sound medical guidance, a family can develop and grow under more favorable circumstances.

## Children In Marriage

All that we have said in this chapter is not meant to imply that children are necessary for successful marriage. Though having children is an important factor in many marriages, some couples cannot or do not choose to have children. On that basis, they can develop quite satisfactory marriage relationships. They may derive satisfactions from companionship, friends, work, and other activities.

---

[7] Elizabeth Ogg, "A New Chapter in Family Planning," *Public Affairs Pamphlet No. 136 C* (New York: Public Affairs Committee, Inc.), 1964.

On the other hand, there are those who believe that having a child can "save" a mismatched or unsuccessful marriage. This is a wrong assumption. Just as marriage does not automatically solve the problems of sexual adjustment, having children does not solve the problems of marital adjustment. The possibility is much greater that an unhappy child will result from an unhappy or broken marriage.

Earlier, we stressed that children are the fruition of the love of man and wife. In mature relationships, they make other contributions to the family. In addition to increasing opportunities for personal interaction and social growth for children as well as adults, children help to broaden the parents' experiences, perspectives, and emotional responses. Responsible parents have greater reason to become more interested and involved in community welfare, education, religion, finance, and politics.

Love, sex, marriage, children, and health do not happen entirely by chance. Fatalistic attitudes or belief in predetermination are philosophical expressions of the helplessness of man and his submissiveness to chance. Our design for attaining and maintaining optimal health is aligned with enlightened self-determination, rational thinking, and the control of choice. Contrary to the abandonment of personal responsibility to "luck" in the lore of romance—which some segments of our culture tend to promote—successful, happy family life is largely a matter of *choice*.

## Problems for Your Consideration

1. What aspects of childhood and early adulthood help prepare for the responsibilities of future parenthood?
2. In what ways does an understanding of the concepts of mental health contribute to preparation for parenthood?

3. Discuss the desirability of family planning and the factors that must be considered to attain it. Name some of the reliable sources of information concerning family planning.

4. What are some of the adjustments that must be made by a married couple who are still attending college when parenthood is "introduced into their lives"?

5. Discuss some of the myths and superstitions which are still prevalent concerning pregnancy and childbirth.

6. What are the factors that have made childbirth safer today than in the past?

## Suggested References

Barnes, Allan C., M.D., "Reducing the Hazards of Birth," *Harpers,* (January, 1964), pp. 31-37.

Calderone, Mary S., M.D., Editor, *Abortion in the United States.* New York: Hoeber-Harper Book, 1958.

Greenblat, Bernard R., M.D., *A Doctor's Marital Guide for Patients.* Chicago: Budlong Press, 1959.

Rostand, Jean, *Human Heredity.* New York: Philosophical Library, 1962.

Rutherford, Robert N., M.D. and Jean J. Rutherford, B.A., *Consultation with Your Doctor for Personal Understanding of Marriage.* Chicago: Budlong Press, 1965.

Stone, Hannah and Abraham Stone, *A Marriage Manual.* New York: Simon and Schuster, Inc., 1953.

# CHAPTER FIVE—*PREVENTING COMMUNICABLE DISEASES*

The prevention and control of communicable diseases depend on a variety of changeable factors creating a need for constant vigilance and research by public health officials, scientists, physicians, and educators. Consider the lack of knowledge about infectious mononucleosis. Though this disease is not highly contagious, some 11 per cent of students who contract it must withdraw from college while recovering and another 4 per cent must reduce their course loads.[1] Medical science has not yet discovered specific measures to either prevent or cure it.

Or consider how disease organisms change. In 1957 the type A influenza virus mutated causing a world wide epidemic of "Asian Flu" because everyone was susceptible to the new strain. Consider how a disease organism such as a staphylococcus, once vulnerable to a specific antibiotic now, has become resistant to it. Thus, the development of new "wonder drugs" must be continuous if medicine is to keep its advantage.

Consider the social changes which influence the incidence of disease within a population. World-wide air travel now can bring diseases such as smallpox and yellow fever to the

---

[1] W. T. Robbins, M.D., "Questions and Answers on Infectious Mononucleosis," (Santa Barbara: Student Health Service, University of California, 1960), p. 1 (Mimeographed).

United States. Or consider the factors that have caused the rapid increase in syphilis in the age group 15 to 25 since 1957. Mass media has exposed this group to many more sex stimuli than comparable age groups in the past; young adults have some knowledge about sex and disease but not enough to be well informed about venereal disease control; sexual behavior has become more permissive; and birth control methods have changed.

An educated public, technical advances, and alert medical and public health personnel are needed to help solve the problems illustrated by these examples. This chapter is designed to help you gain a general understanding of the germ theory of disease, to teach you the basic principles of prevention and control, and to provide you with pertinent facts about some of the diseases with which you may be concerned in the immediate future. Control is better than chance.

## THE DISEASE PROCESS

*Communicable diseases* are illnesses, the specific causative agents of which may pass or be carried directly or indirectly from an infected person or animal to another person. The agents are microorganisms called germs, microbes, or bacteria which are capable of invading the body tissue and causing infections.

An *infectious agent* causes illness by destroying body tissue and/or producing poisons. For example, the spirochete that causes syphilis does so by forming *lesions*, or changes in body tissue. The first of these lesions appears as a pimple which may erode to form a chancre at the point of contact, usually on the external reproductive organs, within ten days to ten weeks. Secondary eruptions show up some four to six weeks later and involve the skin and mucous membranes. A long latent period follows. Then lesions of skin, bone, the central nervous system, and cardiovascular systems develop. The lesions are the result of changes in normal tissue as the parasitic organism lives with the host.

The tetanus bacillus, an organism which can exist in a spore form in soil, is an example of an infectious agent which causes an acute disease by producing a *toxin* (poison). The toxin of tetanus bacilli affects the nervous system of the human being and causes painful muscular contractions, primarily of the jaw and neck and secondarily of the trunk. In severe cases, more complete depression of the nervous system may result in death.

In general, communicable diseases may be considered as having *three stages.* The *incubation period,* the first stage, is the time from exposure until signs and symptoms appear. Knowing the incubation period of a disease is helpful as one can estimate the time range within which a disease may appear after a known exposure. As we have said, syphilis has an incubation period of ten days to ten weeks before the primary lesion appears. Influenza, by contrast, has a short incubation period of twenty-four to seventy-two hours.

The second stage is the *active* or *demonstrable stage.* Cardinal signs and symptoms of inflammation may appear. These are redness, swelling, pain, or sensitivity to touch, fever, and perhaps some loss of function. *Syndromes* (a collection of signs and symptoms) naturally vary with the disease. Some germs attack specific tissue; others are not so particular, and the manifestation of disease depends on the extent of the infection and the tissue or organs involved. For example, the virus which causes infectious hepatitis attacks the liver. Many hepatitis infections are mild and are not readily recognized; others are acute and characterized by fever, nausea, abdominal discomfort, and jaundice. On the other hand, staphylococcus organisms attack many different tissues and have various manifestations that range from a relatively mild single pustule or pimple to a severe pneumonia or to a rapidly fatal blood poisoning. A communicable disease may be *acute* and develop abruptly, as does influenza; or it may be *chronic,* or long lasting, and develop slowly without a specific incubation period, as does tuberculosis.

The third stage is *convalescence.* The disease by this time has run its course and is no longer communicable. Some after-effects may persist, such as weakness or fatigue. One should be careful during this period to avoid complications.

In a few instances, for example, diphtheria and typhoid, the person becomes well but continues to harbor the *virulent* (disease inciting) organisms. This person is then referred to as a *carrier*.

A communicable disease may be sporadic, endemic, epidemic, or pandemic. It is *sporadic* when it occurs at odd intervals and is not persistent, *endemic* when the number of cases within a population remains relatively constant, *epidemic* when there is an unusual number of cases, and *pandemic* when epidemic on a world-wide scale.

There are many types of infectious agents which are known as *pathogenic* (*pathos*, disease; *geno*, producing) microorganisms or disease germs. *Bacteria* include bacilli, cocci, and spirilla. The rod shaped *bacilli* cause tuberculosis, diphtheria, tetanus, and other diseases. Examples of the spherical *cocci* are the staphylococcus which causes boils, the streptococcus which causes sore throats and scarlet fever and the gonococcus which causes gonorrhea. The spirochete that causes syphilis is a spiral shaped bacteria classified as a *spirillum*. *Viruses* are the smallest of pathogens and cause diseases such as poliomyelitis, influenza, and infectious hepatitis. *Fungi* are multicelled microorganisms that cause ringworm and athlete's foot; *protozoa* cause malaria and amoebic dysentery; *rickettsia* cause Rocky Mountain spotted fever.

The cause, or *etiology*, of each infectious disease is difficult to recall, unless you constantly refresh your memory by using the specific term. You should remember, however, that the science of *microbiology*, which includes the study of the etiologic agent, produces the knowledge most necessary for control.

## TRANSFER OF DISEASE

A communicable disease may be *transferred directly* from an infected person or carrier to another person, or from an infected animal to man. Infectious mononucleosis is common to the campus because of dating-kissing practices. Rabies, a disease most commonly encountered in dogs, is contracted directly through the bite of the infected animal. The venereal diseases are almost always transferred through sexual intercourse.

*Indirect transfer* means transmission of disease without close relationship to the infected person, carrier or animal. Indirect transfer is possible only if the organism can survive for a period of time outside the body and some *vehicle* is present to carry this organism from one person to another. For example, it is virtually impossible for syphilis to be transferred indirectly since the organism loses its disease inciting power by drying almost immediately after leaving the body.

There are several vehicles that carry germs. Raw milk may carry streptococci, tubercle bacilli, the agents of undulant fever, and other germs. Water carries viruses, typhoid bacilli, and other organisms that may infect the intestinal tract. Food is a common source of germs that cause intestinal diseases. Soil serves as a vehicle for tetanus and hookworm, and air conveys upper respiratory tract disease organisms. Objects become vehicles when contaminated. Insects such as mosquitoes, lice, and flies serve as vehicles and are referred to as *vectors*. They transfer diseases by inoculation into or through the skin or by deposit of infective materials on the skin or on food.

## NATURAL DEFENSES

If such pathogenic microorganisms are so common, why is it that more of us are not ill? Fortunately, the probability of disease is dependent not only on the numbers and virulence of the germs, but on the resistance of the individual as well. Unfortunately, the *virulence* (disease inciting power) and the number of the germs to which one is exposed cannot be determined, nor can one know if his resistance is high unless he has been recently immunized or has recovered from a specific disease.

General resistance and protection exist physiologically. The *skin and mucous membranes* serve as a line of defense and usually must be broken before germs can enter. Germs in the nose, throat, and bronchi may be trapped in mucus which is expectorated or swallowed and rendered harmless by stomach acids. The *lymph* and *blood systems* protect us when germs penetrate the deeper tissues. Lymph nodes and some of the blood vessels are lined with *phagocytic* (devouring) cells. The blood carries similar phagocytic cells: certain of the so-called *leucocytes* (white cells), that are capable of moving to a point of infection and engulfing and destroying germs. In certain severe infections the "white count" may jump from a normal 6000 per cubic millimeter to 50,000 or more. The liver and spleen have fixed phagocytic cells which devour germs as the blood passes through these organs.

General resistance may be lowered if one becomes fatigued or chilled. Alcohol in the blood stream may retard phagocytosis. Malnutrition impairs the resistance of body tissue. Many diseases such as colds, influenza, and others may weaken resistance so that *secondary invaders* (opportunists) may get a foothold. For example, the virus stage of a cold lasts but a few days, but other organisms already present in the *host* (person infected) may prolong it for a week or ten days.

In addition to general resistance, there is a type of resistance called *immunity,* which is specific against a particular kind of germ. Certain disease organisms stimulate the body to produce chemical substances called *antibodies* that protect one from these specific diseases. If one has such a disease and recovers, he is likely to have developed sufficient antibodies to give him lifelong immunity. This is referred to as a *naturally acquired immunity.* Before they grow to adulthood, most people develop naturally acquired immunities to such diseases as chickenpox, mumps, measles, and German measles. Sometimes a childhood disease appears in such a mild (subclinical) form that it goes unrecognized, yet it produces a high resistance.

## DESIGNS FOR PREVENTION AND CONTROL

Prevention and control of disease are dependent on two basically different designs or approaches. One is to build up the resistance of the individual through specific immunizations; the second is to break the lines of transfer.

The fact that some germs stimulate the production of antibodies makes possible *artificially acquired active immunization, or vaccination.*[2] A vaccine contains the actual disease organisms or their toxins. The virulence and number of the germs or the virulence and amount of toxin are modified and controlled so that the vaccine is sufficient to stimulate the production of antibodies by the person, but without risk to him of contracting the disease. Antibodies are disease specific. For example, the antibodies which the body manufactures in response to the modified smallpox virus do not protect one from the poliomyelitis viruses. The *antitoxins* (antibodies that neutralize toxins) produced by the body in response to the diphtheria *toxoid* (a vaccine made of weakened toxin) do not protect one from the toxin produced by the tetanus bacillus.

You should bear in mind that vaccinations do not necessarily stimulate the production of antibodies sufficiently to produce lifelong immunity. For this reason it is important to receive booster injections at periodic intervals. These intervals vary with each vaccine. In this country, active immunization for diphtheria, smallpox, tetanus, whooping cough, poliomyelitis, and measles should be begun during infancy.

Immunity also can be conferred by injecting into a person immune serums *(antiserums)* which contain antibodies developed in an animal or another person. As the person does not actively produce his own antibodies in this procedure, the immunity that results is referred to as an *artificially acquired passive immunity.* Artifically acquired passive immunizations have definite limitations. Compared with vaccinations they last a relatively short time. Some people become allergic to serum obtained from animals. Unless the serum is administered at the proper time in relation to the time of exposure—which may be hard to determine—it may not be effective. In the case of tetanus, one may be unaware of the injury that provides the portal of entry. Whenever possible, vaccination is preferable. Passive immunity is acquired naturally by the fetus from the mother when antibodies in

---

2 Vaccination is used here in the broad sense to include all procedures to induce active immunity artificially.

her blood stream pass through the placental membrane. These antibodies disappear from the infant's circulation during the first few months after birth.

The following diagram will help you to better understand and remember how the body resists infection.

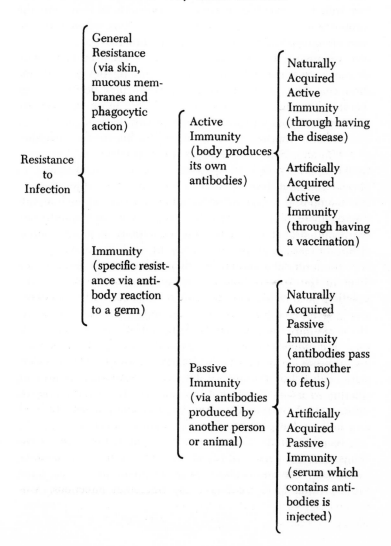

Resistance to Infection

General Resistance (via skin, mucous membranes and phagocytic action)

Immunity (specific resistance via antibody reaction to a germ)

Active Immunity (body produces its own antibodies)

Passive Immunity (via antibodies produced by another person or animal)

Naturally Acquired Active Immunity (through having the disease)

Artificially Acquired Active Immunity (through having a vaccination)

Naturally Acquired Passive Immunity (antibodies pass from mother to fetus)

Artificially Acquired Passive Immunity (serum which contains antibodies is injected)

The second method of preventing disease is by *breaking the line of transfer.* Direct transfer of a disease from man to man or from animal to man can be prevented by isolation and quarantine. In *isolation,* the person with the disease is separated from others. Isolation may be voluntary, as when one tries to prevent others from getting his "flu" by staying away from work, or it may be enforced, as when the law requires a typhoid contact to remain isolated until negative tests for the germ are obtained. In *quarantine,* the movement of the known contact who may be coming down with the disease is limited for at least the incubation period of the disease. This method of control is used only in serious diseases and those about which we have little information.

Indirect transfer can be controlled by various methods of *sanitation.* Sanitary measures are carried out at the community level through the pasteurization of milk, purification of water, insect control, food inspection, and other means. For example, the application of sanitary measures such as the improvement of water supplies, proper sewage disposal and treatment, proper food handling regulations in public eating establishments, and pasteurization of milk have eliminated typhoid fever as a public health problem at the community level in the United States. At the personal level, sanitary practices such as blocking the cough or sneeze with a handkerchief, washing the hands before eating and after evacuation of the bowels, and properly cooking, storing and refrigerating food are important steps in disease control. To illustrate, infectious hepatitis is usually transmitted by personal association. The hands become contaminated with fecal matter at the time of evacuation of the bowels. If a food handler has an unrecognized case, he may transfer the hepatitis virus to food and milk and expose the household to the disease.

In addition to vaccines and antiserums, physicians have drugs that are most helpful in the control and treatment of infections. The *sulfonamides* and the many *antibiotics* have proved valuable in treating many microbial infections. Unfortunately, viruses are, for the most part, resistant to chemotherapy (treatment by chemicals) and antibiotics. Physicians may also use medicines during an infection to support body function or to relieve pain and discomfort. Self-medication for infections is dangerous as it may delay proper diagnosis. When a physician prescribes a drug, he wants to know the physiological condition of the patient, the amount of the drug needed for the nature and degree of the ailment, and the possible side-reactions of the medicine. It was once said the person who has himself for a doctor has a fool for a patient.

## DESIGNS FOR ACTION

Designs for action can best be summarized in the same terminology as the approaches we described for preventing and controlling disease: building the resistance of the individual and breaking the lines of transfer via isolation, quarantine, and sanitation.

You can keep your general resistance high by eating a varied and well-balanced diet, exercising daily, and balancing work, play, and rest to avoid fatigue. Specific resistance must be obtained by immunization. Artificial active immunization procedures should be begun in early infancy and carried on throughout life. Vaccinations for diphtheria, whooping cough, tetanus, measles, smallpox, and poliomyelitis should be completed before the first birthday. Booster injections for diseases vary, but pediatricians and family doctors have recommended schedules which they follow for children of ages one through fifteen.

For the adult, revaccination for tetanus and smallpox is recommended every five years. Recommendations for the schedule of poliomyelitis booster shots have not been determined, but public health authorities advise a booster if an epidemic is imminent. You should keep records of all immunizations, both active and passive. If you are traveling outside of the United States, selective immunizations are recommended or required, depending on where you are going. Vaccines for yellow fever, cholera, typhoid, paratyphoid, typhus, and plague are available.

Voluntary isolation is important to the health of college students. Upon recognizing the common signs and symptoms of infection, you should avoid exposing others during the early stages when the disease is most communicable. As you may realize from your study of this chapter, many diseases start out like the common cold. Your best treatment for the cold is rest during the first twenty-four hours. By staying in your room you provide yourself the best treatment and protect others.

We have already discussed personal sanitary measures that are important in the control of various diseases. You should practice these measures until they become habitual. Too often they are underrated.

Communicable disease control by law is a responsibility of local government and is centered in the Department of Health. As a citizen, you will be interested not only in protecting your own health but also in protecting the health of your community by fighting for and supporting adequate public health measures for communicable disease control.

## CONTROL OF SOME COMMON COMMUNICABLE DISEASES

We have discussed the germ theory of disease, illustrating the basic principles with common communicable diseases. We will now outline some of the infectious diseases, the facts of which should be known by college students.[3]

### Common Cold

1. *Identification:* acute catarrhal infection of upper respiratory tract characterized by inflamed nose and throat. Rise in temperature uncommon. Chilly sensation with runny nose and general indisposition usual. If general indisposition is marked, sometimes the word "grippe" is used. Runny discharge be-

---

[3] Adapted in part from *Control of Communicable Diseases in Man*, Tenth Edition, 1965—an official report of the American Public Health Association, John E. Gordon, Ph.D., M.D., editor.

comes *purulent* (contains pus) later, due to invasion by secondary germs which prolong cold. Spread of the cold to sinuses, lower respiratory tract and middle ear not uncommon.

2. *Cause and transfer:* probably a virus or viruses cause resistance of mucous membrane to be lowered so secondary bacteria get a foothold. Transfer is direct by coughing, sneezing, kissing; indirect by commonly handled and freshly soiled articles.

3. *Prevention and control:* a) keep general resistance high: good diet, avoid fatigue, exposure to chilling, excess use of alcohol; b) no known specific effective immunization; c) protect others, particularly the very young and old, from catching your cold by staying away from them as much as possible. Follow personal sanitary procedures such as covering nose and mouth when coughing or sneezing. Dispose of handkerchief and tissue properly; d) avoid complications by rest during early stages and avoiding violent nose blowing. Children should be taught to wipe, not blow, the nose. Violent blowing tends to spread infection to sinuses and middle ear; e) specific treatment: none; rest during early stages may reduce severity.

## Influenza

1. *Identification:* characterized by sudden onset, fever for one to six days, runny nose, chills, aches and pains in back and limbs, sore throat, and dry cough. Usually self-limiting with recovery in two to seven days. Complications such as bronchitis and pneumonia not uncommon among very young and old.

2. *Cause and transfer:* several different types and strains of virus, some of which have been identified. New types may occur through mutation, as in Asian flu. Few people have immunity to new types, so epidemics occur. Transfer is by discharges from nose and mouth and freshly contaminated articles; possibly air-borne.

3. *Prevention and control:* a) active immunization the only known method. Vaccines for some strains of virus avail-

able, but routine immunization of general population is not recommended; b) personal sanitary measures in relation to coughing and sneezing in close presence of others should be observed. Avoid common use of drinking glasses, towels, and other personal articles; avoid crowds during epidemics; c) specific treatment: none. Sulfonamides and antibiotics not useful if disease is uncomplicated.

### Gonorrhea

1. *Identification:* a purulent discharge of mucous membranes of genital tract. Disease may spread to adjacent or remote tissues, causing acute or chronic processes, among which are arthritis and endocarditis. Frequently causes sterility in both male and female. Detected in the male by noticing discharge from penis and smarting sensation during urination. May go undetected in female during early stages, which are often mild.

2. *Cause and transfer:* gonococcus transmitted in adults by sexual intercourse.

3. *Prevention and control:* a) avoid contacts; b) infection of eyes at birth prevented by adding silver nitrate solution or antibiotic agent; c) specific treatment: antibiotics under medical supervision.

### Syphilis

1. *Identification:* primary lesion (a papule or pimple) which may become an ulcerous chancre at point of entry about three weeks after exposure. Infection without chancre is fairly frequent. The primary lesion is followed about five weeks to as long as 12 months later by mild constitutional symptoms and secondary lesions of skin and mucous membranes. The lesions eventually heal regardless of treatment, but may recur during first five years after infection. Late manifestations of cardiovascular and central nervous systems are among most important affections.

2. *Cause and transfer:* spirochete transferred chiefly through sexual intercourse and occasionally kissing during

secondary stages. Indirect transfer negligible. Prenatal infection of fetus may occur after fourth month of pregnancy.

3. *Prevention and control:* a) avoid contacts; b) specific treatment: antibiotics under medical supervision. Congenital syphilis of fetus prevented by treatment of mother.

### Infectious Mononucleosis

1. *Identification:* fever, enlargement of lymph glands, throat involvement, enlargement of spleen. Fever usually present, but previously mentioned signs may not be.

2. *Cause and transfer:* agent unknown, probably virus. Close contact, person to person, is probable way of transfer.

3. *Prevention and control:* a) keep general resistance high; b) specific treatment: none. If spleen has been involved, contact sports with a risk of injury to the organ should be avoided during convalescence.

### Infectious Hepatitis[4]

1. *Identification:* acute infection characterized by fever, nausea, general discomfort and followed by jaundice. Many infections mild and without jaundice.

2. *Cause and transfer:* virus transferred through intimate person to person contact by fecal-oral route with respiratory spread possible; also transfusion of whole blood from infected person. Epidemics have been related to contaminated food, water, and milk.

3. *Prevention and control:* a) good sanitation and personal health practices such as washing hands in soap and hot water immediately after voiding bowels and always before eating. Keep hands and unclean articles away from mouth. Avoid exposure to spray from mouth and nose. Wash hands thoroughly after handling a sick person or his belongings; b) specific treatment: *none.*

---

[4] Infectious hepatitis and serum hepatitis are clinically indistinguishable. Both may be spread by use of syringes or needles contaminated by traces of blood from an infected person.

### Tetanus

1. *Identification:* characterized by painful muscular con-tractions, first of jaw and neck muscles and then of trunk. Mortality averages about 35 per cent.

2. *Cause and transfer:* toxin of tetanus bacillus. Spores of germ enter through injury, usually a puncture wound. Injury can be so slight that it might go unnoticed. Spore form of bacillus resides in soil.

3. *Prevention and control:* a) active immunization with toxoid beginning in infancy and reinforcing (booster) injection periodically or at time of wound. Vaccination gives protection if injury is unnoticed; b) passive immunity available if person not protected but has disadvantages of allergic reactions for some people; c) specific treatment: tetanus antitoxin and penicillin.

### Tuberculosis

1. *Identification:* primary infection usually "walled off." Slight, if any, signs of it. Occasionally, individual is so run down that germs spread uncontrolled and cause death. Usually a nodule or tubercle forms and remains intact though germs may still remain active.

Progressive tuberculosis: may occur many years after first infection and arise from either individual's walled off bacilli or from bacilli newly received. In former case tubercle breaks down.

2. *Cause and transfer:* tubercle bacillus spread by direct contact and by contaminated articles. Infection usually results from continued and close exposure to a relative or friend as would occur at home or in fraternity or sorority living.

3. *Prevention and control:* a) early diagnosis most im-portant. As there are no early signs and symptoms, case finding through tuberculin tests and x-ray is necessary. A positive test indicates that tuberculosis germs are present in the body. It does not indicate where the infection is located or if it is active or not. Periodic x-ray is therefore indicated

for positive reactors; b) BCG (Bacillus of Calmette and Guerin) vaccine provides partial protection and is used among populations where risk is high. Used very little in this country; b) specific treatment: rest, good diet, drugs, and surgery; c) people with a healed first infection should guard against reactivation by establishing sound health practices.

### Some Common Childhood Diseases

1. *Identification:* many childhood diseases begin with signs and symptoms similar to the common cold, with a rash and swelling appearing later. As there are no effective vaccines for German measles, mumps and chickenpox, and complications with the first two may be serious for adults, it is best for children to have these diseases and acquire immunity naturally. German measles may endanger development of fetus if contracted during first trimester of pregnancy; mumps may involve reproductive glands of both male and female if contracted after puberty.

2. *Cause and transfer:* Many of these diseases due to virus infections which are transferred person to person. Childhood diseases highly communicable.

3. *Prevention and control:* a) all infants should be vaccinated for whooping cough, diphtheria, smallpox, poliomyelitis, measles, and tetanus. Child's physician will recommend a vaccination schedule which begins at two months of age and includes booster injections through age fifteen; b) specific treatment: varies with the disease. Medical care should be sought.

## Problems for Your Consideration

1. What is a sensible immunization program for the young adult? Under what circumstances might rabies, typhoid, and Rocky Mountain Spotted Fever immunizations be recommended?
2. How often should one be tuberculin tested? X-rayed?

3. What common misconceptions are there regarding the prevention and treatment of the common cold?

4. As prospective parents, what should you know about immunization schedules for infants and children?

5. How do local health departments attempt to control the following diseases: syphilis, smallpox, rabies, and typhoid?

## Suggested References

Abramson, Martin, "V.D.—Return of an Old Scourge," *Today's Health.* 38 (December 1960), p. 50.

Anderson, Gaylord W., Margaret G. Arnstein, and Mary R. Lester, *Communicable Disease Control.* New York: The Macmillan Company, 4th ed., 1962.

Beck, John, "Mono: The Medical Mimic," *Today's Health.* 43 (February 1965), p. 36.

Carpenter, Philip L., *Microbiology.* Philadelphia: W. B. Saunders Co., 1961.

Cooley, Donald G., "Viruses: Molecules That Cause Disease," *Today's Health.* 40 (February 1962), p. 23.

Hilleboe, Herman E. and Granville W. Larrimore, *Preventive Medicine.* Philadelphia: W. B. Saunders Co., 1959.

Smith, Geddes, *Plague on Us.* New York: The Commonwealth Fund, 1941.

# CHAPTER SIX—*CONTROLLING NONCOMMUNICABLE DISEASES*

Far too often the attitude, "I couldn't care less," is reflected in the reaction of the young adult when conditions such as heart disease and cancer are mentioned. Actually he ought to care *more!*

The young adult who is in college is generally in a good state of fitness. Although all of his campus habits of living may not be optimal, especially in terms of adequate rest and nutrition, he has the opportunity to establish habits that may actually *prevent* heart disease and other noncommunicable diseases later. Too often his immediate desires so overshadow his long term goals that, without realizing it, he is overlooking the possible current choices that could prevent serious difficulties later.

Noncommunicable diseases can and do occur in the college-age person. Asthma, rheumatic heart disease, allergies, and epilepsy, just to mention a few, are health problems with which college students live. College students also die from diseases of this noncommunicable type. Of the five leading causes of death of the fifteen to twenty-four-year age group, malignancies are the second and heart disease is the fifth most common cause. The two combined, however, account for less than one-fourth of the total deaths caused by the first place leader, accidents. Homicide and suicide occupy the third and fourth places in such a ranking. Statistics also indicate that as collegians grow older, noncommunicable diseases begin to play a more prominent part in morbidity and mortality data. Thus, *now* is the time to ascertain what *you* can do to make yourself less susceptible in the future!

This chapter is organized around six "designs for action," rather than only the basic facts and terminology of specific diseases. Many of these diseases develop slowly over a period of time; often it is possible to detect this gradual development early in its course. Hopefully, these designs will help you recognize some of the skills, understandings and patterns that *you* can establish now for possible protection and control of noncommunicable disease later. The designs are:

1. Maintaining a desirable weight, exercise, and recreation program.
2. Accepting the challenge of controlling normal stress and tension.
3. Acting on the facts regarding cigarette smoking.
4. Recognizing possible symptoms or danger signals.
5. Exercising intelligence concerning periodic medical examinations.
6. Considering inherited tendencies.

The noncommunicable conditions which we shall discuss in this chapter are given various categories or titles in today's literature. They are called chronic, chronic progressive, degenerative, diseases of adults, diseases of older persons and even the "big killers." Each disease we shall mention fits at least one of these categories. But all of them fit the category of the *noncommunicable* disease. None is caused by an infectious agent or can be transferred directly to another person. All will affect you directly or indirectly, however. Because heart disease and cancer are the two leading causes of death for all persons twenty-five years and older, the chances are that you, some members of your family and some of your friends may die or suffer from one or the other. It is estimated that "somewhat over two-fifths of the population of the United States have some chronic condition, but in only a fraction of the cases does the condition impose a limitation of activity . . . . More than one-sixth of the population under age 15 and two-fifths of the people at 15-44 years have at least one chronic disease."[1]

It seems important, therefore, for us to be aware of specific habits or patterns that we can *establish* or *break* now, since the positive health we have tomorrow may be the result of what we choose to do today.


## DESIGNS FOR ACTION

The following six *designs for action* are behavior patterns which you can establish now in an attempt to gain protection against the effects of some of the noncommunicable diseases.

### I: Maintaining desirable weight and exercise programs

For many collegians, their weight in college is the weight they should continue to maintain throughout adulthood. Generally speaking, the more weight that is gained by young adults, the more they become susceptible to specific noncommunicable diseases. The more we weigh the more we demand of our *cardiovascular* (heart and blood vessels) system.

A study by the Society of Actuaries reveals that today the average man gains eleven pounds between the ages of twenty-five and forty; the weight pattern for women shows little gain until after the age of forty-five.[2]

Physiologically, weight control is primarily a matter of acquiring and maintaining eating habits in which you consume daily only the amount of food containing the number of calories which you will burn daily. Calories are the units of energy found in all foods. If you eat more calories than your

---

[1] Metropolitan Life Insurance Company, "The Prevalence of Chronic Conditions," *Statistical Bulletin* (September 1963), pp. 3-5.

[2] Metropolitan Life Insurance Company, *Overweight—Its Significance and Prevention* (New York: One Madison Avenue, 1960).

body can use in its normal daily activity, the excess is stored as fat. The extent to which the calories are burned is determined primarily by the amount of exercise you take and the basal metabolism rate. (This rate represents the energy expended to maintain the essential physical and chemical processes.) Most people who live moderately active lives need approximately 15 calories per pound to maintain a desirable weight. The person who wants to maintain a 150 pound weight should consume approximately 2,250 calories daily. The less active a person is the fewer calories he needs to maintain optimal weight.

For most individuals a program of moderate, daily exercise is equally as important as calorie counting. The role of exercise in weight control can be overlooked and underestimated. Walking instead of riding, going up and down stairs instead of going up and down in elevators, plus maintaining a leisure time recreational program of some active sport are highly recommended after you leave the campus as well as now.

You can select a daily diet containing a variety of foods which represent specific portions of the four major food groups (milk, fruits and vegetables, meat, bread and cereals) to include a greater or lesser number of calories, whichever you desire. In toto, the recommended number of servings of the four major food groups contain all the nutrients needed daily by an individual. Eating patterns which consistently contain food selected according to both nutrient value and caloric content are far superior to crash diets which are diets maintained for a short period of time. Weight lost by crash diets is generally regained because the old eating habits have not been changed and are quickly resumed.

To the layman, the term *overweight* represents a weight of five to ten percent over the desirable number of pounds while the term *obesity* indicates an excessive accumulation of fat in the body. Obesity in most individuals is due to overeating although some cases may be due to a glandular malfunction. Sometimes this overeating is caused by psychological factors; a physician must then determine whether the psychological factor itself is best treated by simply tolerating the obesity or undertaking a reducing program. The psychological aspects of obesity sometimes favor abandoning a reducing program in some individuals in order to maintain psychological effectiveness.

Reasons why collegians gain weight after graduation are varied. One of the most common, however, is continuing college eating habits while discontinuing college exercise habits. Proper weight control demands a check and balance system between how much you eat and how much you exercise. Thus, exercise habits play a vital role. As a student you may walk, run, climb steps, and exercise recreationally far more than you realize. If you change these exercise patterns after you leave the campus, so also then should you change your eating patterns. Regular, moderate exercise is a must for healthy individuals who desire to maintain optimal weight and positive health. And those individuals who pursue it through recreational activities and sports may be gaining more than exercise for the sake of exercise and weight control!

Obesity is definitely a predisposing or contributing factor to atherosclerosis, heart attacks, and strokes. "Obesity is reported to precede diabetes in 85 per cent of the cases and is considered by some to be second only to heredity as the most activating factor in its development."[3]

Scientists are trying to determine the exact role played by diet and exercise in *atherosclerosis,* the most common form of *arteriosclerosis* (hardening of the arteries). Atherosclerosis is a type of arteriosclerosis that involves a thickening that narrows the inside opening as well as a hardening of the walls of the arteries. This is due to slowly forming deposits of fatty materials on the inner lining. Most serious cardiovascular disorders are partially caused by the process of atherosclerosis.

In recent years, the substance *cholesterol,* a fatlike, pearly substance which adheres to the inner walls of the arteries and

[3] United States Department of Health, Education and Welfare, *Diabetes Source Book,* Public Health Service Publication No. 1168 (Washington, D.C.: Government Printing Office, 1964), p. 23.

thus narrows, irritates, and damages them, has been a source of much controversy among medical scientists as a cause of heart disease. A diet that is high in the saturated fats as found in meat and dairy products is thought by some to raise the cholesterol level; individuals with a lot of cholesterol in their blood tend to have heart attacks earlier in life than others. However, the cholesterol level varies a great deal with exercise, the drugs that a person may take, his eating patterns, and even his emotional tension. Since many factors besides the quantity of foods and fats that are consumed are evidently important in regulating the cholesterol level, it is suggested that the safest path to follow at the present time is to eat all types of food fats in moderation.

*II: Accepting the challenge of controlling normal stress and tension*

Stress and tension are normal and to be expected as a part of our daily lives. Undoubtedly our stresses today are no greater than those of our grandparents or great-grandparents; they are simply a different variety. Thus it behooves us to learn to live with stress and to deal with it constructively. As a college student you "asked for" many kinds of stress situations when you decided to work for a baccalaureate. In this process, you have recognized that stress can produce different effects, physically and mentally. You know that certain kinds of tension can literally raise your blood pressure. Emotional upsets increase the work load of your heart. The individual with hypertension (high blood pressure) attempts to anticipate stressful situations and, by keeping them under control, also helps to control his hypertension.

The exact role of stress on the heart, on disease in general, and on the other parts of the body has not been absolutely determined. However, there is an interaction that can be harmful in certain situations. Stress may be a contributing but not a direct cause of both ulcers and heart attacks. Thus, the person predisposed to conditions such as ulcers, hypertension, and heart attack has a definite need of the ability to deal with and control tension.

Since there is no specific "test" to tell us if we are susceptible, all of us are involved automatically in stress control. Change of pace is important; the ability to relax is important; the role of adequate sleep and rest cannot be stressed enough. The individual who consistently burns the candle at both ends may be asking for more anxiety than he can handle. Much tension and anxiety cannot be reduced or eliminated, but it can be anticipated and kept under control! This "design" was emphasized in Chapter Two, also, since the control of stress is so vital to both psychological and physical effectiveness.

*III: Acting on the facts regarding smoking*

The effects of cigarette smoking on health have been given wide publicity. Regardless of whether you currently do or do not smoke, you need to be aware of these data as they relate to the noncommunicable diseases. Facts do speak for themselves in many ways; what these facts say to you is, to a large extent, your choice of what you *want them to say!*

The increased incidence of lung cancer which parallels the increased consumption of cigarettes strongly indicates evidence of a causal relationship between the two. Clinical, bio-statistical, and laboratory research also indicate evidences of this causal relationship. The protective mechanism known as the ciliary cleansing mechanism of the bronchial tubes apparently is vulnerable to cigarette smoke, and its function is impaired by it. The extent of this impairment is determined by the number of cigarettes smoked daily, the amount of inhalation and the duration of the smoking. Lung cancer seems to be rare in persons who have never smoked, except for those who by occupation have had extensive contact with radioactive ores, chromates, nickel, and carcinogenic gases from the burning of gasoline. "In comparison with non-smokers, average male smokers of cigarettes have approximately a nine- to ten-fold risk of developing lung cancer and heavy smokers at least a 20-fold risk."[4] (The heavy smoker

---

[4] Advisory Committee to the Surgeon General of the Public Health Service, *Smoking and Health* (Washington, D.C.: Government Printing Office, 1963), p. 31.

is characterized as the individual who smokes at least a pack of cigarettes a day.) Such rates diminish for men who have given up smoking. Cigarette smoking is found, also, to have a causal relationship to cancer of the larynx; a similar relationship between pipe smoking and oral cancer appears to have been established. Data also suggest an association between cigarette smoking and cancer of the esophagus and cancer of the urinary bladder.[5]

Of equal significance to the cigarette-lung cancer data are these excerpts cited by the Advisory Committee to the Surgeon General in the publication, *Smoking and Health:* "Cigarette smoking is the most important of the causes of chronic bronchitis in the United States. . . . A relationship exists between pulmonary emphysema and cigarette smoking . . . for the bulk of the population in the United States, the importance of cigarette smoking as a cause of chronic bronchopulmonary disease is much greater than that of atmospheric pollution or occupational exposures . . . male cigarette smokers have a higher death rate from coronary artery disease than non-smoking males, but it is not clear that the association has causal significance . . . epidemiological studies indicate an association between cigarette smoking and peptic ulcer which is greater for gastric than for duodenal ulcer.[6]

Excessive cigarette smoking has been cited as a factor which is predisposing to arteriosclerosis, heart attack, and stroke.[7] The American Heart Association has also publicized the fact that the heart attack death rate is 50-150 per cent higher among heavy cigarette smokers.[8]

Although the majority of the research studies have used men as subjects, there is no evidence to indicate that women who smoke are affected in a different manner.

---

[5] *Ibid.*, p. 32.

[6] *Ibid.*, pp. 31-32, 39.

[7] Louis N. Katz, M.D., Samuel A. Levine, and others, *A Statement on Arteriosclerosis—Main Cause of Heart Attacks and Strokes* (New York: National Health Education Committee, Inc., 135 East 42nd Street, n.d.).

[8] *The American Heart*, X, No. 3 (Summer, 1960). Published by the American Heart Association and its affiliates.

The overwhelming evidence points to the conclusion that smoking—its beginning, habituation, and occasional discontinuation—is to a large extent psychologically and socially determined . . . cigarette smoking is a health hazard of sufficient importance in the United States to warrant appropriate remedial action.[9]

*IV: Recognizing possible symptoms or danger signals*

An awareness of symptoms or danger signals seems to be almost too simple to be of such vital importance. The danger signals which have been most widely publicized are those by the American Cancer Society that *may* mean cancer. These include:

1. Unusual bleeding or discharge.
2. A lump or thickening in the breast or elsewhere.
3. A sore that does not heal.
4. Change in bowel or bladder habits.
5. Hoarseness or cough.
6. Indigestion or difficulty in swallowing.
7. Change in a wart or mole.

The American Cancer Society frequently reminds us that none of these danger signals is a *sure* sign of cancer. When conditions such as coughing, indigestion, and unhealed sores persist for no apparent reason longer than two weeks, then they need to be investigated. Some types of cancer have no early signs and, unlike many diseases, pain is seldom an early cancer signal.

*Malignant* (cancerous) conditions develop when, for unknown reasons, healthy cells lose their normal function and begin to multiply in an uncontrolled manner.

Malignant tissue has the distinct ability to break away from the original site after an undetermined amount of "localized" growth and to start new growths or colonies in

---

[9] Advisory Committee to the Surgeon General of the Public Health Service, *Smoking and Health, op. cit.,* pp. 40, 33.

other parts of the body. *Benign* or noncancerous tissue also grows, but it always remains attached to the original site and does not have such "break-away" power. The detaching of malignant tissue and its colonization in other parts of the body by means of the blood and lymphatic systems are termed *metastasis.*

As a malignant growth develops, it slowly invades and breaks through the surrounding tissue, lymph, and blood vessels causing seepage or discharge and minor bleeding. Such seepage and minor bleeding may be detected in some cases and become a signal indicating an abnormal condition. Thus, some internal cancers may be indicated by blood appearing in the sputum, urine, or feces. Many cancers originate on the surface of a tissue such as the skin or uterus or the lining of the mouth; therefore, their presence is often readily detectable. Cancer of the larynx usually can be detected early because even the smallest growth on the vocal cords produces hoarseness.

The Papanicolaou ("Pap") test, in which a sample of the cells normally shed by the uterine lining is obtained easily and painlessly, and the monthly breast self-examination may produce evidence early enough to make a cure possible. Women are particularly fortunate in this respect since cancer of the breast and uterus are the leading sites of cancer in women in the age group of fifteen to thirty-four years.

In *leukemia,* which is cancer of the blood-forming organs, metastasis takes place immediately; there is an overproduction of white blood cells which not only fail to carry out their disease fighting functions but also infiltrate other tissues and organs. Another similar type is lymphoma or *Hodgkin's disease,* which begins in the lymph glands and spreads through the body's lymph channels. Leukemia and lymphoma are the leading kinds of cancer in men ages fifteen to thirty-four.

Although some drugs are helpful in controlling and retarding the growth of malignant cells, none has been found that will destroy them. Physicians rely on surgery and radiation to cure cancer, and if such therapy is to be successful, it must be instituted before metastasis occurs. Thus, discovery of a malignant condition prior to metastasis is essential.

Knowledge and recognition of danger signals are ways of helping yourself discover possible malignancies and also possible *diabetes*. The diabetic lacks enough of the hormone *insulin* to properly utilize the sugars and starches in the diet. In the process of excreting this excess sugar, an extra load is put on the kidneys because an excess of water is also excreted. This explains the cause and effect relationship of two of the common danger signals of diabetes: excessive thirst and frequent urination. Hunger is another by-product, since the caloric energy usually provided by the sugars and starches is lost. Additional symptoms are tiring easily, losing weight, itching, and slow-healing infections. Not every diabetic experiences such definite symptoms; some are simply not functioning up to par. Perhaps this explains why medical statisticians estimate that 50 per cent of the cases of diabetes in this country are undiagnosed. Most individuals with diabetes are fortunate because control can be attained by diet, or diet plus medication and exercise. The diet is adjusted to the specific needs of the individual. Diet alone is satisfactory for some while others require diet plus medication (insulin) which is administered by injection or taken as an oral compound. The form of insulin is dependent upon the severity of the condition. Exercise is important for all diabetics since it improves the ability to use sugar.

Some types of *heart disease* also have warning signals.

Uncomfortable breathlessness or exertion, persistent palpitation with only mild effort; pain under the breast bone which may radiate from the middle of the chest into the shoulder and down the inside of the arm . . . however, these symptoms may occur for reasons other than heart disease. Indigestion can produce symptoms which are very similar to those of heart disease. Sometimes the symptoms are almost impossible to tell apart. However, indigestion is much more common . . . shooting pains near the heart can be due to many causes, most of which are not serious.[10]

---

[10] American Heart Association, *Questions and Answers About Heart and Blood Vessel Diseases* (New York: 44 East 23rd Street, 1963).

*Angina pectoris* is the term applied to the pain that appears to emerge from the breast bone and often is the result of a lack of sufficient blood flow to the heart muscle. When we use the term heart disease, we are actually referring to many different conditions that affect the heart and circulatory system. A more accurate term is cardiovascular disease.

Another condition which first occurs more often in childhood than adulthood is *rheumatic fever*. Although this disease is difficult to diagnose, there are some warning signals such as fever, pain or inflammation in the joints (often miscalled "growing pains"), failure to gain weight, paleness, poor appetite, fatigue, repeated nosebleeds, and St. Vitus' dance. Rheumatic fever generally follows a streptococcus infection of the throat, nose, or tonsils. The inflammatory condition of the joints may be temporary, but if the heart becomes involved, then the disease develops more serious aspects and is known as *rheumatic heart disease*.

We cannot overstress that all of these symptoms may mean conditions other than the ones we have designated here. But neither can we overstress that they mean that something is not up to par and a physician should be consulted.

*V: Exercising intelligence concerning periodic medical examinations*

Undoubtedly no one piece of advice is offered quite as often as "If . . . see your physician." Probably one's age is a determining factor in how frequently one goes to a physician just "for a check-up." Usually, the college-age student is not concerned with conditions which have no symptoms or are unsuspected. The periodic medical examination is not important to him except for specific reasons such as marriage or the requirement of a job application. This is understandable now, but it will not always be so. As one grows older, the medical examination assumes great importance. Often the physician's routine examination will disclose a possible difficulty that is in an early stage and without visible symptoms. For example, the routine testing of the urine might reveal a possible diabetic condition; routine x-rays could show possible heart or lung difficulties. Likewise, the periodic dental examination could disclose periodontal diseases, nutritional insufficiency, or malignancy.

Most noncommunicable diseases which are discovered early can be helped, and many can be cured or controlled. For example, rheumatic fever could be eliminated if streptococcal infections such as "strep sore throat" were properly and promptly treated; likewise rheumatic heart disease may be prevented if rheumatic fever is diagnosed early and properly treated. The possibility of cancer of the prostate gland, a disease with few early symptoms and a leading cause in the cancer mortality statistics of older men, should be checked by a physician periodically. The same applies to cancer of the colon and rectum.

Physicians can also help control most types of cardiovascular disease that are detected early. Some of the most common types besides atherosclerosis are heart attack, hypertension, strokes, and rheumatic heart disease.

A *heart attack* which is also termed *coronary artery disease*, occurs when a section of the heart muscle is deprived of blood. This may be caused by the clogging of a coronary artery due to atherosclerosis or a blood clot *(thrombus)*. Heart attacks are more common in men than in women. The attack is generally followed by a healing process which is facilitated by a detour system *(collateral circulation)* set up by the smaller arteries to feed the portion of heart deprived of its original supply.

*Hypertension,* or high blood pressure, is sometimes termed a symptom rather than a disease, per se. When a person's blood pressure remains higher than it should, an effort should be made to determine the cause. Many times, a specific cause cannot be found and the individual learns to live "in moderation" with this condition.

*Strokes* occur when the blood supply to a portion of the brain is reduced or eliminated. The portion of the brain affected loses its ability to function, causing paralysis or loss of vision, hearing, speech, or other functions. Causes of such conditions may be a blood clot or hemorrhage. Terms used for various kinds of strokes include cerebral thrombosis, cerebral vascular accident, and cerebral hemorrhage.

Rheumatic heart disease is the result of the scarring of the valves of the heart due to an allergic inflammatory reaction to the rheumatic fever infection.

It is obvious that a physician, through the periodic medical examination, may be able to detect, diagnose, and determine the extent and seriousness of conditions such as these. Early detection makes possible the use of the continuing advances in treatment and prevention of cardiovascular disease.

It is futile to worry about symptoms that may or may not be heart disease or cancer. You would undoubtedly urge your parents to have a yearly check-up for the purpose of "early discovery," or "just to be sure." Likewise, such a habit formed *now* by *you* may mean that you will attain adulthood in a state of positive health. Surely young men and women in their early forties, at the prime of their family and vocational responsibilities, are grateful that they avoided some hazards by realistic long-term planning started in college.

Perhaps a word of caution is in order here regarding the medical quack. He finds his best customers are those people with chronic or long continued conditions such as some types of cancer, circulatory disorders, and arthritis. Only a licensed physician can give you reliable information—beware of the individual who promises or guarantees any kind of cure or control. Such a control may *seem* to work, since many noncommunicable diseases pass through stages of inactivity or dormancy which can be mistaken for improvement or even cure. This is especially true in many kinds of arthritis and rheumatism, and the quack takes advantage of such cycles in this type of condition. As well as taking a cancer patient's money under false pretenses, the cancer quack also deprives this person of any possible medically accepted treatment.

## VI: *Considering inherited tendencies*

"Forewarned is forearmed." Diabetes occurs five times more frequently among blood relatives of diabetics than among other people. Thus the person who has a parent or grandparent who is or was a diabetic seeks medical advice periodically on ways he might avoid this condition. Such a person also checks carefully into the family history of a potential marriage partner, so that he may evaluate the possibility of diabetes in their children.

*Predisposition* to a disease is the same as saying there is a physiological tendency toward that disease. This tendency may be an inherited one which may or may not express itself during one's lifetime. The circumstances which can reveal or trigger into expression this susceptibility may often be anticipated and often avoided.

Inherited susceptibility to several of the noncommunicable diseases is known. Besides diabetes, these include epilepsy, pernicious anemia, asthma, and other allergies, ulcers, cancer—and possibly some of the cardiovascular diseases, particulary atherosclerosis.

You cannot change your heredity, but you can attempt to control some of its factors and lessen your chances of acquiring certain diseases. Surely one way to do this is by periodic medical examinations.


Undoubtedly, you already have lived and, indeed, will continue to live the rest of your life with noncommunicable diseases that do not appear in lists of major causes of death for people of your age group. Most common perhaps is *allergy* in its multiple forms; this is a hypersensitivity to specific types of foods, plants, cosmetics, pollens, medicines, animals, or dust to which the body reacts. These reactions vary and may include rashes, nausea, difficulty in breathing, headache, and inflammation of the mucous membranes. Hay fever, asthma, skin disorders, and digestive disturbances are specific types of illnesses which are a result of a reaction to an *allergen*. Many allergies can now be controlled by means of vaccines and chemotherapy. Still others are outgrown during adolescence.

Young adults who have had rheumatic fever or rheumatic heart disease should be aware of the danger of subsequent streptococcal infections since another "repeat" strep infection could do further damage. Thus, protection against and prompt, proper treatment of a recurrent infection is of utmost importance.

Today's young adult who suffers from epilepsy or convulsive seizures often can keep them under control by means of anticonvulsive drugs. Seizures are a result of irregular brain waves and they occur in a variety of forms, the most severe of which is known as the *grand mal;* the *petit mal* is the more mild form. It is well to know that a person having a grand mal seizure should be protected from injuring himself; during a seizure a soft object such as a rolled handkerchief should be placed between the teeth and the person should be placed on the floor or the ground away from stationary objects. A deep sleep generally follows a severe seizure. The misconceptions that the epileptic is mentally retarded or incapable of leading a happy, productive life need to be erased. What the epileptic needs most in our society today is understanding, acceptance, and an opportunity to show that he *can* be a productive citizen.

You as a young adult can begin to develop patterns now to protect yourself against many of the noncommunicable diseases. The six designs for action in this chapter are, essentially, choices which you may either make or disregard. The value you place now on such factors may well play a large part when, at the age of thirty-five or forty, in your role as a parent, a community leader, and a business or professional man or woman, you will be eager "to live most and to serve best." Making the right *choices* now may reduce some *chances* later!

## Problems for Your Consideration

1. Some of the noncommunicable diseases are not considered possible to *cure*, but, rather, just to *control*. Identify these and their forms of control.

2. Rheumatic fever and rheumatic heart disease are mentioned in several of the chapter's "designs for action." Consider in detail the relationship between the two and its significance to you.

3. The use of cigarettes is a multi-faceted problem. Discuss the psychological and social implications that are involved in the decision "to smoke or not to smoke."

4. Many noncommunicable diseases such as muscular dystrophy, multiple sclerosis, and cerebral palsy are not mentioned in this chapter. These, like many other noncommunicable conditions, are not found among the leading causes of death, yet they are highly significant health problems. Can they be cured? Can they be controlled?

5. How do health organizations such as the American Cancer Society and the American Heart Association contribute to the control of the various noncommunicable diseases?

## Suggested References

American Heart Association, *Questions and Answers About Your Heart and Blood Vessel Diseases.* New York: The Association, 44 East 23rd St., 1963, 26 pp.

Arthritis and Rheumatism Foundation, *Arthritis Explained.* New York: the Foundation, 10 Columbus Circle, 16 pp., n.d.

Conklin, Groff, *Diabetics Unknown.* Public Affairs Pamphlet No. 312, New York: Public Affairs Pamphlets, 22 E. 38th Street, 1961, 27 pp.

Johns, Edward B., Wilfred C. Sutton, and Lloyd E. Webster, *Health for Effective Living.* New York: McGraw-Hill Book Company, Inc., 3rd ed., 1962, Chapter 12.

McGrady, Pat, *Science Against Cancer.* Public Affairs Pamphlet No. 324, New York: Public Affairs Pamphlets, 22 E. 38th St., 1962, 20 pp.

# CHAPTER SEVEN—*RECOGNIZING THE CHALLENGE OF COMMUNITY HEALTH*

In the previous chapters we have discussed a number of the health concerns of the 1960's that have particular pertinence for the college student. The actions of individuals in relation to each of these areas will, to a large extent, determine the degree of effectiveness which will characterize their lives. Health is *not* just a matter of chance. We have discussed many of the *choices* that you, as an individual, need to consider.

Some problems in the health area, however, are most effectively handled by *groups* of individuals. Problems such as air pollution, radiation, and water pollution are matters of individual concern that are simply too extensive to be solved by individual action alone. We need community, state, and perhaps even national efforts to solve problems like these. Such group efforts do *not* lessen the importance of the individual. His decisions, his vote, his financial support, and his understanding of the significance of such problems make his role an extremely important one, though slightly different from the one we have previously discussed.

With all of the advantages of modern living, can it be possible that some of our health problems are, indeed, a result of modern living—modern community living? The answer is yes. We cannot avoid considering the price of such progress, and whether the advances represent a significant rise in the level of our civilization. Our understanding of these problems and our individual choices and group actions in relation to them will determine, in a large measure, the type of life that we enjoy in our communities.

## RADIATION: MIRACLE OR MENACE?

At first glance scientific advances do not always appear advantageous. Radiation consists of the energy from the nuclei of atoms of certain physically unstable elements. It can cause cancer. It can supply energy for war. Such a potential causes our government and its citizens much concern. But radiation also has many useful and highly beneficial aspects. Its good is the hope, and its evils the despair, of this era.

### Radiation's Benefits

On the "plus" side of the ledger are many advantages to man that have come as a result of the use of radiation. We are familiar with the benefits of an annual chest x-ray and periodic dental examinations. There is no need to be concerned about the body's exposure to this amount of radiation. Aside from the use of x-rays for diagnostic medical and dental purposes, artificially produced *radioisotopes* (radioactive elements) are used for both diagnosis and treatment. The progress of these radioactive drugs can be traced in the body, thus enabling the physician to measure blood flow, study the functioning of the digestive system or a specific organ or gland, or carry out other diagnostic procedures. Radioisotopes can suppress the activity of certain tissue or destroy diseased tissue, and can often be made to act more selectively than x-ray radiations. For example, the functioning of an over-active thyroid gland can be reduced, sometimes eliminating the need for surgery, or seeds of a radioactive material can be implanted in a tumor to destroy it, while causing little if any damage to surrounding tissue.[1] In addition, radiation can be beamed to cancerous tissue from outside the body, as with x-rays or radium. Methods have been developed to protect healthy skin and tissue while the diseased tissue is receiving this radiation.[2] With attention to all necessary safeguards we can continue to receive the benefits of radiation without risking injury.

### Radiation's Possible Dangers

The possible adverse effects of radiation upon man are varied, and their severity is related to the *amount* of radiation received, the *extent* and particular *part* of the body radiated, the *age* of the individual, and the *frequency* of radiation. Estimates have been made by scientists of the possible adverse effects that might occur from various exposure levels. It has been suggested that these include an increase in the number of cases of leukemia and some other forms of cancer, anemia, abnormalities of pregnancy, sterility, and various genetic effects.

Overexposure to the sun or to fire can be dangerous. So, too, can overexposure to radiation. But the chances of receiving an overexposure to radiation are slight. Persons who work with it are cognizant of its potential dangers and take the necessary precautions. The controlled and proper use of radiation for medical purposes is not a cause for concern, and the nuclear test programs at the present time involve

---

[1] Squibb Medotopes Service, *Radioactive Medicine* (n.p., Reissued, June, 1962), pp. 7-12.

[2] United States Department of Health, Education, and Welfare, *Treating Cancer—Surgery, Radiation, Chemotherapy* (Washington: Government Printing Office, 1960), p. 7.

health risks so slight that any counter-measures are believed unnecessary.[3]

## Man and Radiation

Man always has been exposed to some radiation. Natural sources consist of energy from the sun as well as from radio-active materials naturally present in the earth's crust, in water, and among the elements that constitute man himself. These sources have given man relatively little cause for worry, but with the advent of man-made radiation more interest and concern have been demonstrated. Testing programs of nuclear weapons and radiation from medical sources probably have been subjected to the most intensive questioning.

The biological effects of radiation depend upon the amount of energy which the tissues absorb. This is measured in terms of RAD or Radiation Absorbed Dose, which is a measure of the energy imparted to matter by ionizing particles per unit mass of the irradiated material. (The term Roentgen may be a more familiar one. This refers to the absorption of gamma rays only; RAD includes alpha, beta, and gamma rays.) In man's lifetime he probably receives ten RAD from natural radiation sources. A chest x-ray taken with the usual type of automatic equipment gives an exposure of about 0.3 RAD, and as far as is known, this is harmless. Stomach or intestinal x-rays give an exposure of 15 or 20 RAD, but this, too, is a relatively small amount.

Since exposure to radiation at any level may be a risk to health, it is recommended that individuals and their physi-cians keep records of their medical and dental exposures and avoid unnecessary exposures. The advantages that the average person gains from his necessary exposures to man-made radia-tion (about 85 per cent of which are medical ones at this

---

[3] Federal Radiation Council, *Estimates and Evaluation of Fallout in the United States from Nuclear Weapons Testing Conducted Through 1962, Report No. 4* (Washington: Government Printing Office, 1963), pp. 25-26.

time) are, however, believed to far outweigh any possible disadvantages.

## Protection From Radiation

In spite of radiation's many advantages, there still remain questions in the mind of the average citizen: How can I protect myself from present low levels of fallout that may contaminate fruits and vegetables? Are our milk supplies endangered by fallout? Will the next generation be damaged by the radiation we are receiving now? To all of these questions there are reassuring answers. Neither food nor milk supplies are receiving sufficient radiation from fallout that would suggest that any dietary changes should be made.[4] In addition, the present and anticipated levels of fallout are not believed to constitute an undue risk to the genetic future of the nation.[5] Dangerously high levels of fallout would be detected rapidly by the Division of Radiological Health of the United States Public Health Service. Its surveillance networks all over the country determine current radiation levels in our environment—air, water, milk, and food.

Whenever possible hazards are discovered, it is customary to attempt to discover ways in which protection from them can be obtained. Persons who work with radioactive materials use protective clothing, and the regulation of exposure time and shielding to protect the body from exposure are also used. Some particularly interesting approaches to protection have been research to discover drugs that will reduce radiation's biological effects[6] and a process for removing radioactive strontium from milk.[7] Further research in these areas and others is being carried on.

Is exposure to radiation a cause for concern? No—not at present levels. At the present time man has a choice:

---

[4] *Ibid.*

[5] *Ibid.,* p. 25.

[6] "Anti-Radiation Drug," *Science News Letter,* 81 (April 7, 1962), p. 222.

[7] "Removing Radioactive Material from Milk," *Public Health Reports,* 80 (March, 1965), p. 219.

to make use of radiation's benefits, which far outweigh its dangers, or to neglect the use of one of science's most useful and beneficial tools.

## MAN AND MACHINE: FRIENDS OR ENEMIES?

More people, more cars, more highways, more speed—and more *accidents*—have resulted in what some experts call the number-one lifesaving challenge in America today.

The modern car is, indeed, one of man's most pleasurable and highly prized scientific developments. Like other pleasures, the auto also has its price, and that is the staggering injury and death toll on our highways. Does this slaughter and maiming have to exist? Perhaps a look at some of the factors believed to cause accidents will help answer that question. It is estimated that approximately 85 per cent of auto accidents are caused by the actions of the drivers themselves.[8] Mechanical defects of the car, bad weather, and poor road conditions do cause some accidents, but these factors are believed to be of relatively minor significance. The driver and his emotional state are considered of major significance. Faulty attitudes and judgment and poorly controlled aggressiveness and competitiveness are prime factors in the accident picture.

In 1963 the National Safety Council indicated that speeding, drinking, disregarding stop signs, or violating the law in other ways contributed to 98 per cent of fatal accidents.[9] Why? According to research studies, driver *attitude* is the most important factor in the driving situation. Attitudes, linked with man's emotions, are a part of his personality, and, therefore, of his habitual behavior. So man tends to drive as he lives—either impulsively, aggressively, showing lack of respect for authority, or cautiously, with foresight and consideration for others. It is worthy to note, however, that even the most cautious and considerate individual can become a

---

[8] A. E. Florio and G. T. Stafford, *Safety Education*, Second Edition (New York: McGraw-Hill Book Co., Inc., 1962), p. 178.

[9] National Safety Council, *Accident Facts* (Chicago: The Council, 1964), p. 48.

victim of his emotions, and therefore become temporarily "accident-prone." The student worried about the exam he is about to take, the mother whose young children have been raising havoc all afternoon in the house, the young person who has just broken up with his girl or boy friend—these are all people who take their problems behind the wheel with them, giving less than full attention to the job of driving. Combine any situation of this type with a wet highway or some other environmental hazard and the already "accident-prone" person is in an "accident-prone" situation, thereby increasing the probability of an accident.

Obviously, the accident situation has far-reaching personal ramifications. It is also a problem of considerable community and national importance. Over 40,000 persons are killed annually on our highways, and the number of persons injured is estimated to be as high as one and one-half million. Auto accidents are the major accident problem of the college age young person and are, in addition, the major cause of death for the child and young adult population, with over 14,000 deaths during 1963 in the five to twenty-four age group.[10] The economic impact represents a loss of billions of dollars to our nation, but it is not easy to convert into dollars and cents the loss incurred by a family that has had one of its members killed.

### It's Your Choice!

What can be done about the accident problem that plagues our communities and our nation? Driver education, highway improvements, safer car designs, more strict traffic law enforcement, and more severe penalties for law violation are all factors in the picture. We noted earlier, though, that the vast majority of auto accidents are caused by the *drivers* themselves. That clearly puts the responsibility on each one of us.

Perhaps the well-known but insufficiently-heeded alcohol question is worthy of discussion at this point. Choices arise

---

10 *Ibid.*, p. 60.

once again. Will you drink? If you decide "yes," you should recognize and act appropriately upon the significance of the relationship between drinking and accidents. Special studies conducted in various states indicate that as many as 50 per cent of accidents involve a drinking driver.[11] Alcohol is properly classed as an anesthetic, and depending upon the amount consumed, can have a pain relieving, quieting, or sleep producing effect. Though some people appear noisy and excited during and after drinking, this type of behavior really indicates the *depressant* or slowing-down action of alcohol upon the nervous system. It is difficult to state the *exact* effects that a certain amount of alcohol will have on any person. It depends on the person's size, whether he is drinking on an empty stomach, what he is drinking, the time over which the drinking is extended, and a variety of other factors.

We can say with certainty, however, that *any* amount of alcohol has *some* effect on the nervous system and, therefore, on one's ability to drive and make the necessary judgments and reactions. Research studies indicate that a blood alcohol concentration of 0.05 per cent (about 2-3 drinks) impairs the driving ability of most individuals, and some are seriously impaired at this level. Most state laws recognize that individuals are *legally* "under the influence" at a concentration of 0.15 per cent and above. However, it cannot be assumed that the accident problem will not arise until one is legally "under the influence of alcohol." The "had-been-drinking" driver is a real highway menace. He is the one who *thinks* he is in fine condition, not realizing (or not admitting) the dangers to which he is subjecting himself and others. The choice he makes here may involve a matter of life or death.

At the present time the automotive seat belt is believed to be the most effective single item of protective equipment available, since it keeps you in your seat, inside the car, and thereby reduces serious and fatal injuries by at least one-third. Being thrown from an auto or against a windshield greatly increases the chances of death or injury. Because belts are

---

[11] *Ibid.*, p. 52.

easy to get into and out of, there is no reason to be concerned that they might trap the car's occupants and prevent their escape from a burning or submerged vehicle. Less than 1 per cent of accidents causing injuries are in this category, and seat belts are *still* good protection, as they improve a person's chances of remaining conscious. Since a majority of traffic deaths occur within 25 miles of one's home, and at speeds of less than 40 miles per hour,[12] the college student needs to use seat belts in driving on the campus and in the nearby community, as well as when driving home for the weekend via the freeway. With continued acceptance of this already available safety device and an increase in the individual driver's use of it, something *can* be done about auto accidents.

### THE FLUORIDATION STORY

One further choice that you may be called upon to make concerns the *fluoridation* question—or, as it is frequently termed, the fluoridation *controversy*. Millions of persons are fortunate to live in areas where the water supply is naturally fluoridated, (fluoride is in the ground and the water absorbs it), but millions of others are being called upon to make a choice that will affect the health of children and adults in their communities.

As many as sixty years ago a possible relationship between dental *caries* (decay) and low-fluoride amounts in the diet was demonstrated in England. Many communities in the United States have been drinking *naturally* fluoridated water for years, and studies of tooth decay and tooth loss clearly indicate that the people in these communities have fewer cavities than those in comparable but nonfluoridated areas. Similar results are noted in studies made in communities which have added fluoride to their water. Children, whose teeth are developing, benefit most from fluoridation programs, but recent research begins to indicate that adults may also

[12] National Safety Council, *Seat Belts Save Lives* (Chicago: The Council, n.d.), pp. 1-6.

gain in an equally beneficial way. Fluoridated water seems to effect a strengthening of bones in older people, making them less likely to fracture in case of a fall.[13]

Is there a need to be concerned about the dental decay problem in the United States? In school examinations, dental defects lead the list of those uncorrected, and an extremely high percentage of children suffer from dental decay. This untreated problem frequently carries over into adult life, and it is estimated that by the age of 40 dental decay and other dental conditions have caused approximately one-fourth of the people to lose all their teeth. Even the average college-age person has had at least a dozen cavities filled. Here, indeed, is an area where individuals, in their communities, can choose to take advantage of preventive dental care which will lessen the need for costly restorative dentistry.

What complicates this seemingly simple and clear-cut situation? There are individuals who question whether drinking fluoridated water may increase the incidence of heart disease, cancer, and other conditions. Other opponents claim that fluoridation is mass medication and that no one should be forced to use medication in which he does not believe. Both of these arguments can be answered. Communities that have been drinking naturally fluoridated water for years have been investigated and no higher rates of cancer, heart disease, or other conditions have been found there than have been found in comparable communities drinking nonfluoridated water.[14] When the mass medication accusation is considered, it is interesting to recall that most people eagerly buy milk that has been fortified with Vitamin D and bread made with enriched flour. These additions to our food help improve diets and health. Why has the addition of fluoride to water, to improve dental health, had such a difficult time being accepted by many persons? Misunderstanding and misinformation are

---

[13] Frederick J. Stare, "References in the Literature Indicating that Fluoride Favors the Deposition of Calcium in Bone" (March, 1964), (Mimeographed.)

[14] "Fluoridation . . . The 65 Per Cent Answer to Tooth Decay," *Ohio's Health*, 13 (January, 1961), pp. 18-19.

two of the factors which have affected the way in which community members have voted on this issue.

The facts are simple. Health authorities recommend a concentration of one part of fluoride to a million parts of water as an effective deterrent to tooth decay. Many persons drink naturally fluoridated water that contains many times this amount and suffer no ill effects. However, if the concentration is excessively high over a long period of time, mottling of tooth enamel may occur. Normal water purification technology would readily prevent such a high level in artificially fluoridated water treatment processes.

Fluoridation of public water supplies is an inexpensive procedure, averaging about ten cents per person per year. More than 2700 communities and 48,000,000 people in the United States are drinking water that has had fluoride added to it. This procedure has been recommended by all the major health organizations in the United States, including the American Medical Association, the American Dental Association, and the United States Public Health Service. The decision—or the vote—may be yours someday.

## OUR WATER PROBLEMS

Outdoor recreation has become one of the most popular types of family activity in recent years, and our state and national parks and recreational areas are being used to capacity in most areas of the country. In fact, their capacity is being taxed heavily. Herein arises one of our major community and national problems. The water sports enthusiasts, interested in fishing, swimming, boating, or water skiing, are discovering that in many areas their opportunities for such activities are curtailed, due to the impurity or the lack of available water.

When we talk about water, we need to recognize that the problem is having the *right amount,* at the *right place,* at the *right time,* and of *usable quality.* This is a problem that affects our everyday life, regardless of our interests or where we may live. In many cities, beaches and picnic and boating areas are becoming less attractive and less safe for use. Miles of streams are being lost each year for fishing, and millions of fish are being killed, due to *pollutants*. Many of our local rivers and streams are bubbling with detergent foam, and in many cities drinking water is becoming less palatable because of the chemicals that must be added to control the pollutants in the water supply.

It is reliably estimated that by the year 2000, water needs will have reached crisis proportions. What is the cause of this impending danger? It's as simple as addition and multiplication and, indeed, that is exactly what it is. Our growing population, 180 million in 1960, is expected to reach 260 million by 1980. The more people there are, the more water will be needed and desired for living. Our communities are requiring more water for household and recreational uses, and water of suitable quantity and quality simply is not available.[15]

More important, however, than *city* and *agricultural* water needs, is the tremendous increase in water use by *industry*. This use currently is over 160 billion gallons per day, and by 1980 it is estimated that this figure will more than double.

A further problem is created by the vast array of new products and chemical substances that have been developed in recent years. The wastes which accompany their production are difficult to handle, but the greater problem is *disposing* of the products after they have been used. Detergent wastes, pesticides, and other products may end up in our drinking water and in our recreational water areas, and using present procedures it is difficult to remove these substances.

We do not have enough "new" water to meet the needs of modern living and modern industry, and water has to be *used over again*. In some areas it is used as many as four times as it flows into a river and passes along from city to city. Water reuse can be hazardous. There are serious questions as to whether present water purification processes

---

[15] United States Department of Health, Education, and Welfare, *Focus on Clean Water*, Public Health Service Publication No. 1184 (Washington: Government Printing Office, 1964).

remove or inactivate viruses. These considerations will become even more important if future water needs require more reuse of water for human consumption.

## Is There a Choice?

The major responsibility for the cleaning up of its waters rests with the local community. Federal funds have been available since 1956 to assist local governments in financing sewage treatment facilities, and states and the federal government can both bring legal action against those responsible for polluting waters. Industries, which are partly responsible for the pollution problem, are studying ways to develop useful products from their wastes, and means of disposal which will not cause pollution. We need to develop improved procedures for reusing water in industry and conserving water in both agriculture and industry. We also need to construct many more sewage treatment plants. Scientific endeavor, which has helped to create water problems, is also being used in the solution of them. All of us, as homemakers, manufacturers, consumers, voters, and taxpayers, have important roles to play, and must become more aware of the severity of the problem.

## THE AIR WE BREATHE

A serious and more visible community problem is that of *air pollution.* This is not a new problem, but it has become increasingly more serious as our industries and cities have become larger and as automobiles, a chief source of pollutants, have become more numerous. Fortunately, it is a problem that recently has received some very necessary attention. But more is required. It is estimated that 90 per cent of our urban population lives in areas having air pollution problems, but air pollution control programs exist in very few of these communities.

More factories, more people, more houses, more cars, and, in brief, more activity have resulted in an increase in the dust and other pollutants which fill the atmosphere. In recent years, we have given more consideration to the value of better air, as an accompaniment of better living. We now realize that smoke and other pollutants need *not* fill the air we breathe.

What are these pollutants and where do they come from? Dusts, gases, chemicals, smoke, soot, and others are among the trouble makers. They are not all visible, and some cannot be smelled, so it is very possible to be unaware of their presence, and to believe that the air in one's own community is not polluted. An understanding of the sources of pollutants is necessary for comprehending the dimensions of the problem: *Industrial* and *commercial* sources, ranging from steel mills to small dry-cleaning plants, provide a significant portion of an area's pollutants. *Municipal* sources such as burning dumps, heating plants in schools and other buildings, and road maintenance equipment create further pollutants. *Household* sources include heating systems for homes and apartments and trash burning, while *transportation* sources of pollutants include autos, trucks, buses, ships, and locomotives.

If all cities were located in areas where the wind blew all the time, air pollution might be of considerably less significance. *Weather* and *geography* play an important role in the dimensions of this problem. Cities in river valleys or surrounded by mountains are more likely to have air pollution problems. In such physical circumstances, meteorologic conditions accentuate the trapping of cooler air in the valley, with relatively warmer air above it. The pollutants are likely to be trapped over the cities by these masses of warmer air which have risen and act like the lid on a kettle, preventing the pollutants from escaping. When this *temperature inversion* occurs, and lasts for days at a time, the pollutants accumulate and severe "smogs" develop.[16]

There is evidence that air pollution is harmful to man's health. Although eye irritation is well-known to those who live in the Los Angeles area and in some other major metro-

---

[16] United States Department of Health, Education, and Welfare, *Air Pollution—A National Problem*, Public Health Service Publication No. 975 (Washington: Government Printing Office, 1962), p. 11.

politan districts, the principal hazard appears to be damage to the respiratory system. The cumulative effects of breathing polluted air over a period of years are hard to observe and document, however. A strong relationship between the occurrence of bronchitis and emphysema and long-time residence in areas where there is air pollution has already been demonstrated.[17] Certain heart diseases and some types of cancer are more numerous among city dwellers than among rural people. Other studies are concerned with the possible relationship between lung cancer and air pollution, since a number of pollutants have been shown to produce cancer in experimental animals.[18] Positive evidence showing air pollution as a *direct* cause of disease is not plentiful. It is believed, however, that it is one of the many factors producing chronic bronchitis and other respiratory diseases.

Less difficult to evaluate are the dramatic, severe, and relatively rare air pollution "episodes," such as those occurring in Donora, Pennsylvania in 1948 and in London in 1952 and 1962. In Donora a thermal inversion occurred over the city and the smog did not lift for several days. Approximately 6000 persons were reported ill and 20 persons died. Most of those who died were elderly people who already had heart and lung disorders, but many young and apparently healthy persons were made ill. There is research evidence indicating that those who were seriously affected by this "episode" were sick more frequently afterwards and died sooner than their neighbors who were present but unaffected by the smog. Future research into the health effects of air pollution is indeed challenging and needs the active support of an informed public.

These health effects, serious though they may be, are not the only problems of significance. Many pollutants are harm-

---

17 Eric C. Cassell, "Polluted Air and Health," *National Tuberculosis Association Bulletin* (January, 1965), pp. 11-13.

18 United States Department of Health, Education, and Welfare, *The Health Effects of Air Pollution,* Public Health Service Publication No. 640 (Washington: Government Printing Office, Rev. 1959), pp. 4-5.

ful to agriculture and yields may be reduced or the quality of the products affected. These losses are reflected in the higher prices for agricultural products that the grower is forced to charge. From the purely personal standpoint, air pollution is both annoying and expensive, and the effects of pollution on one's feeling of well-being cannot be ignored.

There does appear to be sufficient evidence to warrant an intensive attack upon the problem of air pollution, although all of the scientific answers to the problem are not known. Without such an attack, air pollution problems will increase in the years ahead as our population grows and still greater industrial development takes place. Some industries have taken leadership in acquiring equipment that will cut down on the smoke and gases that are discharged into the air. Many large cities have air pollution control agencies associated with the local health department and attempt to regulate citizen and industrial activities, such as open burning, that contribute to the problem. Since the automobile is now recognized as a major cause of air pollution, it will probably not be too long before "blow-by" devices, to cut down on exhaust fumes, will be standard equipment on all new cars.

When at least seven billion dollars of loss are suffered annually from the effects of air pollution, it seems incongruous that the national total expenditure at the local level for air pollution control is approximately eight million dollars (and more than half is spent in California). The further development of community programs for air pollution control is urgently needed now. Progress will come only when people are willing to work and pay for improvement. The air pollution menace may not impress itself upon the population as forceably as others, but it *is* dangerous and costly.

No community has to work alone in attacking this problem. In December, 1963, Congress enacted Public Law 88-206, the Clean Air Act, which provides for a national program for the prevention and control of air pollution. If people care— and *act*—an effective air pollution control program can be designed for any community.

## OUR COMMUNITY HEALTH ORGANIZATIONS

All of the health concerns that we have discussed in this chapter and the previous ones have some effect upon us as individuals. To think that their effects stop at this point would be short-sighted indeed. There is little that happens in modern life that affects only *one* individual or one family. For this reason, our governments at the national, state, and local levels have been concerned for many years with the health of citizens.

The Constitution of the United States makes no specific provision for health, so the broadest power to protect the public health has fallen to the states. The states in turn have delegated power to the local departments of health. State health departments have advisory, policy making, coordination, and regulatory functions. They might assist a community that has a sudden outbreak of a communicable disease, or develop standards for the licensing of health and medical personnel in the state or work with a community which is attempting to establish a community-wide mental health program.

Organization for health is needed at the community level to meet adequately the health needs of a particular locality. A few years ago when you went to a local church or high school to "drink" your Sabin polio vaccine, you were participating in a program coordinated by your *local* health department. Its many functions may include provision of maternal and child health clinics, keeping of vital statistics on births, deaths, and illnesses, communicable disease control, health education programs, visiting nurse services, enforcement of sanitary standards, and a variety of other activities. It is indeed unfortunate that these services are too often minimal in many localities because of inadequate financial support. The local board's health regulations help protect the health of all community members.

Federal health powers are related to interstate and international problems and health factors which concern the promotion of the general welfare of the nation. The various government agencies that are most directly concerned with the people's health are under the jurisdiction of the Department of Health, Education and Welfare. One of the largest of these agencies is the United States Public Health Service, whose varied functions include research, consultative services, and the granting of funds for special health programs and research work. Although the Service operates a number of hospitals, including two for narcotics addicts, and one for patients with Hansen's disease (leprosy), the majority of its work is not the provision of medical care to individual patients. The Service's National Institutes of Health constitute the nation's largest health research agency and, as such, make invaluable contributions to the health of the people of this country and others. These health organizations at the local, state, and national levels are known as *official* agencies. They are tax supported.

The *voluntary* health organizations are characteristically American. A multitude of health groups have developed, each focused on a particular health need or problem. The American people have recognized specific needs and have accepted the responsibility for doing something about them. Many of these "voluntary" agencies are well-known to the average citizen. The American Heart Association, the American Cancer Society, the Arthritis and Rheumatism Foundation, the National Association for Mental Health, and others conduct programs of research, education, and service in relation to their particular interests. Such organizations are dependent upon our financial generosity and voluntary participation to continue their work.

A typical organization of this type will spend a large proportion of its budget for *research* to discover new knowledge concerning its particular field. Its *education* program may include the production and distribution of pamphlets and films to improve the understanding of the public, scientific meetings for physicians and health personnel, and the provision of speakers for school and community groups. Many of the agencies offer direct *services* to patients and families of those afflicted. Assistance in the form of social counseling, home care education, and rehabilitation services may be provided. Each organization, depending on its particular focus and decisions made at the local level, has its own variation of this plan.

There are, at the present time, at least two problems that are related to the voluntary health agencies. The first problem is recognized by those who are asked to support the organization's work. Almost every possible disease or health condition appears to have one organization, or several, working in its behalf. The voluntary contributor is almost constantly being asked for money. Where shall he give his support, since he obviously can't give to all groups? In most communities the organization of a Community Chest or United Fund has assisted in the solution of this problem, but a number of these voluntary organizations still do not wish to give up their successful fund raising programs. A second problem—if it can be called a problem—is that science has succeeded in controlling some of the conditions which these organizations are concerned about. Always looking to the future, and toward total health and better living, some of these groups have simply changed or broadened their emphases. The National Foundation for Infantile Paralysis, now the National Foundation, is focusing on birth defects and other crippling conditions. Although tuberculosis is not yet completely conquered, the National Tuberculosis Association is also giving consideration to other respiratory conditions. Hopefully, this situation, caused by scientific advances, will continue and the voluntary organizations will continue to meet the challenges of the future.

In some communities there is a third problem: the duplication and overlapping of services and functions of the various health agencies. Voluntary and official agencies have grown rapidly since the turn of the century. Freedom of our people, their aggressiveness in meeting problems, economic well-being, and decentralized responsibilities for health in government provided a fertile field for independent as well as rapid growth. This growth has, however, created some problems related to overlapping of functions, duplication of effort, imbalance of programs in meeting needs, and methods of financing public health. To solve some of these problems there has appeared a relatively new health agency, the *health council*. The council is made up of representatives from medical and dental professional societies and citizen's groups as well as executives from voluntary and public health agencies. The health council may be organized on a county, city, or metropolitan basis. Its purposes are to promote the coordination of public and voluntary health work, to analyze community health problems through special studies, and to serve as a forum for discussion of future policies and plans to protect public health.

We have discussed only a few of the community health problems that make living in the 1960's a challenge. Your awareness of the problems, concern about them, and willingness to cooperate in their solution with your local, state, and national health organizations will contribute to better health and better living for you, your community, and your nation.

## Problems for Your Consideration

1. In what ways can an *individual* contribute to the control of air and water pollution problems?
2. Discuss the scientifically substantiated pro's and con's in the water fluoridation controversy.
3. What routine use of x-rays should be a part of every adult's personal health program?
4. What is the significance of the modern concept of the accident-prone person?
5. Have the services of any voluntary health agencies ever benefitted you or your family? How?

# Suggested References

Carter, Richard. *The Gentle Legions.* Garden City, New York: Doubleday and Co., Inc., 1961.

Chambers, Leslie A., "Fresh Air or Foul?" *Journal of Health, Physical Education, and Recreation.* 32 (December, 1961), pp. 29-31.

Dublin, Louis I., *Water Fluoridation: Facts, Not Myths.* New York: Public Affairs Committee, Inc., 1957.

Hanlon, John, *Principles of Public Health Administration.* St. Louis: The C. V. Mosby Co., 3rd ed., 1960.

United States Atomic Energy Commission, *Health Aspects of Nuclear Weapons Testing.* Washington: Government Printing Office, 1964.

United States Department of Health, Education, and Welfare. *The Struggle for Clean Water.* Public Health Service Publication No. 958, Washington: Government Printing Office, 1962.

————, *What About Radiation?* Public Health Service Publication No. 1196, Washington: Government Printing Office, 1964.

# CHAPTER EIGHT—*SPENDING THE HEALTH DOLLAR WISELY*

One of the dilemmas faced by the American consumer is how to spend his health dollar *wisely*. There are many choices! Do you know how to make them? Are you aware of the *real* value and the potential dangers of some of the prominently displayed "health" products on today's market? Do you realize that the work of many organizations and agencies is directed toward helping to inform and protect you from fraudulent products? Do you know how to distinguish the well trained and ethical physician from the "quack" practitioner—and how to choose a physician? Have you considered the different types of health insurance that are available, and your present and future needs for protection from the high costs of medical care?

We have written this chapter so that you may become more aware of the many choices that you can make in spending your health dollar wisely, and so that you will have the understandings upon which you can base wise choices.

### HEALTH PRODUCTS: TRUE OR FALSE?

Many of the products and services we hear of today direct their advertising toward the known values and interests of the consumer. This is, indeed, good business and it has proven as successful in the health area as in any other. In our society there is considerable emphasis on good looks, good grooming, youthfulness, and other similar traits. Consequently, the "be young and good looking" approach can easily gain a foothold, and it provides a lucrative market about which the intelligent consumer should be realistic. Wrinkle removers, hair growing tonics, miracle formula skin creams, royal jelly, and other products claim to be fountains of youth for those who are not as young as they wish. Will any of these products restore lost youth? Not likely. Skin creams and lotions may soften the skin, but any claims beyond that are false. Wrinkles and baldness? When they appear, they are here to stay. Any confidence placed in products that claim otherwise is *misplaced*. Dependence upon recommended practices of healthful living, rather than upon highly advertised but questionable health products, is still the most effective way to look your best.

If overweight or obesity is keeping you from being your best, there are many products that can help you (if you believe all you hear and see!) These products, among the most popular on the market, ignore the known fact that to reduce satisfactorily you have to decrease your calorie intake, increase your activity level, or both. No pills, wafers, or miracle treatments can do it for you—it takes will power, diet control, and medical advice to be sure you are dieting safely. All that results from the use of these highly advertised products is possible danger to the health of the user and a useless expenditure of money (to the extent of one hundred million dollars annually).

A second approach geared to modern thinking might be called the "better-to-be-safe-than-sorry" philosophy. In more scientific terms it might be thought of as preventive medicine, but exactly what it *really* prevents is highly questionable. This category of products includes the *food fads* and *vitamin supplement* preparations. The vitamin question can be settled quickly: the majority of nutrition authorities agree that unless your physician prescribes special vitamin preparations, there is no need for the average person to supplement his diet with these products. Some people, due to illness or other conditions, need additional vitamins; but the physician is the one best qualified to determine this, not the individual himself. A well balanced diet supplies more than enough vitamins to fulfill normal body needs.

The food fad question is an involved and interesting one. The food faddist may think he has a product of great value and want to share it. However, he may be an individual who is interested only in making money. Whatever his reasons, he usually has a good sales pitch and an armload of testimonials to assist him in selling food supplement plans or special foods that he claims have therapeutic values. The food huckster may promote his products by public lectures to which community members are invited, or he may be a door-to-door salesman who attempts to diagnose your ills and sell you something for what ails you. Human nature is, in a sense, one of his best allies. Who hasn't felt tired or depressed recently? Who doesn't want to have more pep and energy? The faddist plays on these desires and fears in order to sell his products. He also plays on our ignorance, and uses a combination of scientific sounding mumbo jumbo and confusion to make us question the little we may know about the science of nutrition.

These merchants of menace promote a number of nutrition myths as they attempt to sell their products:

1. The *soil depletion* myth. According to the faddists the soil is so poor that foods grown on it are nutritionally inadequate. There is no scientific evidence to support this claim. Crop yield per acre may suffer from poor soil, but food value does not.

2. The *overprocessing-of-food* myth. Some food processing techniques and cooking methods reduce the nutritive value of food. The food faddist tries to capitalize on this fact by selling various types of cooking utensils, food

supplements, or "natural" foods. What he ignores is that vitamins and minerals, in regulated amounts, are added to flour, bread, milk, and other products to improve their nutritional adequacy. In addition, he seems ignorant of the fact that the once-prevalent nutritional deficiency diseases, such as rickets and pellagra, are almost non-existent today.

3. The *subclinical deficiency* myth. *Subclinical* means that there are no symptoms, that there is no evidence of disease, and that the condition cannot be detected. According to the faddist, however, that "tired feeling" indicates the condition exists, and that the faddist's products will cure it. The logic of associating a tired feeling or other aches and pains with a subclinical deficiency is highly questionable.

4. The *disease causation* myth. According to the faddist, most diseases are due to faulty diets. Heart disease, cancer, arthritis, and other diseases can all be prevented (or cured) by using the faddist's products. Reliable scientific evidence indicates otherwise. And if use of the faddist's products keeps the individual from seeking medical attention, the results can be tragic! Poor nutrition *can* cause lowered resistance, fatigue, and irritability, and there *are* diseases caused by poor diets, but they are almost unknown in the United States today.

It seems hard to believe that anyone really believes these myths or any of the many other claims that food faddists make. It is conservatively estimated, however, that the cost of vitamin and "health food" quackery is five hundred million dollars a year. Quackery is big business.[1]

A third approach made by the health hucksters might be termed *pseudo-scientific.* In this truly scientific era it is not surprising that our normal interest in and dependence upon scientific developments should be capitalized upon by these

---

[1] George P. Larrick, "Report on Quackery from FDA," *Proceedings, National Congress on Medical Quackery,* October 6-7, 1961 (Chicago: American Medical Association, n.d.), p. 13.

quacks. Their ozone generators, Depolaray, Spectro-Chrome, radioactive ore, and other scientific-sounding apparatus have been accepted, unfortunately, by many unknowing persons. Many sufferers from arthritis, rheumatism, and cancer are among their clients. In the arthritis field alone it is estimated that two hundred and fifty million dollars annually has been spent for unproven, misrepresented products in vain attempts to obtain relief. Some of these products, such as alfalfa tea, honey and vinegar, and various ray machines, are pure quackery. Others, such as vibrators, though not entirely useless, are misrepresented and lead the sufferer to expect results far beyond what is possible.[2]

Cancer quackery is similarly widespread. The Hoxsey Cancer Clinic in Dallas is an example of note. It existed for over thirty years, charging exorbitant fees for pills and other medicines. The National Cancer Institute and the Food and Drug Administration proved that its medications were worthless and could find no verified cures of cancer. Other clinics of this type have been known, as well as an estimated 5000 individual cancer quacks.

It is easy enough for those of us who are in good health to ridicule the use of worthless products and the patronage of unqualified practitioners. To the person in ill health, particularly the one who has a disease or condition for which modern science has not yet found all the answers, the quack and his nostrums offer a promise that is quickly accepted. The quacks flourish, bringing cures to none and delaying or preventing others from getting the treatment that might make the difference between life and death. The various agencies and organizations that attempt to control quackery are numerous, but most effective control is accomplished when intelligent consumers are alert and on guard against these serious threats to their health.

Many of these products and services are advertised in very carefully chosen terms. Modern advertisements are so

---

[2] Ronald W. Lamont-Havers, "Quackery in Arthritis," *Proceedings, National Congress on Medical Quackery,* October 6-7, 1961 (Chicago: American Medical Association, n.d.), p. 51.

clever that even the most intelligent consumer can sometimes be fooled. Before too long a time has elapsed the unsuspecting consumer accepts what he sees and hears, almost unquestioningly. The use of such products gets into the realm of self-medication, and when proper treatment for any condition is postponed, the outcome may be unfortunate.

To protect yourself against the ads that ask, "Do you always feel tired?" or "Does your back ache after working all day?", ask yourself the following questions:

1. Are the facts stated in clear, simple language without resort to confusing technical terms? (Long "scientific" terms may be used to impress prospective buyers.)
2. Are the claims acceptable in terms of good common sense and logical reasoning? (The thinking consumer will not be convinced by holes burned in handkerchiefs, the amount of fizz produced by a tablet, or the like.)
3. Does the advertisement play upon common fears, dread of disease, or superstitious beliefs? ("Have you got tired liver?" or "It could be your kidneys" would be examples of such scare techniques.)
4. If research is cited to prove a point, was the research conducted by an unbiased scientific organization? (A manufacturer's department, for example, could be biased.)
5. If research is cited to prove a point, were the findings published in recognized medical or dental journals? (State, regional, and national periodicals of the health professions and others approved by them.)
6. If opinions of scientific authorities are cited to support a statement, are these persons identified by name, position, place of residence, and professional standing? ("Scientific authorities agree that . . ." sounds impressive but means nothing.)
7. Are the scientific authorities cited in support of a particular point properly qualified in terms of that specific issue? (Competency in one field does not necessarily carry over into another.)
8. Are the statements made approved or accepted by professional medical, dental, and public-health associ-

ations? (If you aren't sure on items 1-7, check with
the medical society or your health department.)[3]

There is no doubt that evaluation of health products and
advertising will save you money. It might also save your life.

## Agencies That Help to Protect Our Health

Even the most intelligent consumer needs the additional
protection offered by several government agencies. Particularly noteworthy are the activities of three agencies: the Food
and Drug Administration, the Federal Trade Commission, and
the United States Post Office Department.

*The Food and Drug Administration.* The Food and Drug
Administration's work consists of activities to protect the
consumer by insuring that (1) foods are safe, pure, and wholesome, (2) drugs and therapeutic devices are safe and effective,
(3) cosmetics are safe, (4) all of the aforementioned are
honestly and informatively labeled and packaged, and (5)
certain hazardous household cleaning agents, paint removers,
wax, etc. carry adequate warning labels.[4]

To carry out its many activities the Food and Drug
Administration receives appropriations from the federal government and fees for the testing of drugs and the establishment of safe tolerances of pesticides and colors allowed in
foods. This is a very large scale operation. In addition to
its Washington headquarters the FDA has eighteen field
district inspection offices and laboratories and forty-one resi-
dent inspector posts throughout the country. Its staff consists
of approximately 3000 employees. Some idea of the volume
of the agency's activities can be appreciated by knowing that
during a recent year FDA's activities included:[5]

---

[3] Fred V. Hein, "Evaluating Health Advertising," *National Education Association Journal*, 49 (January, 1960), p. 57. Reprinted by
permission.

[4] Food and Drug Administration, *FDA, 1963* (Washington: Government Printing Office, 1963), p. 1.

[5] United States Department of Health, Education, and Welfare,
*Annual Report 1963* (Washington: Government Printing Office, 1964),
p. 332.

Making 36,639 inspections of food, drug, and cosmetic
factories

Collecting and testing 87,729 samples of products produced
in the United States (foods, drugs, cosmetics, hazardous
substances)

Making 146 inspections involving the illegal sale of pre-
scription drugs

Making 104 inspections to check on quackery practices of
lecturers

Making 26 inspections to check on radioactivity

Making 14,695 inspections involving food additives

Completing court action on 290 Federal court cases

Certifying batches of antibiotics, insulin

Receiving and clearing requests for the marketing of new
drugs

A more specific account of some of its activities gives
an indication of the protection being given by the FDA. The
promotion and nationwide sale by mail-order of a "cancer
cure" was halted by a Federal District Court ruling. The
product contained wheat, salt, yeast, and water, sold for
$6.75 to $10.00 per half-ounce (a one-week supply) and was
claimed to dissolve tumors and act as a tonic and a panacea
for all kinds of diseases and conditions. As a hope-giving
treatment it could, of course, cause damage to persons who
delayed seeking competent medical care until they were
beyond help.[6] In 1962 one of the FDA's best known and
most dramatic actions was its prevention of the sale, in the
United States, of the birth deforming drug *thalidomide*. These
examples illustrate only two of the agency's many activities
that protect the consumer's health. Clearly, this protection
is needed.

In making all of its seizures and inspections the FDA is
enforcing the Food, Drug and Cosmetic Act and five other
consumer-protection laws. In addition, the FDA controls the
marketing of new drugs by requiring manufacturers to submit

---

[6] United States Department of Health, Education, and Welfare,
*FDA Report on Enforcement and Compliance* (Washington: Government
Printing Office, March, 1964), pp. 7-8.

evidence of safety and effectiveness and the adequacy of manufacturing controls. No new additive may be used in or on foods until the promoter submits to the FDA evidence of its safety when tested on animals.[7]

*The Federal Trade Commission.* The Federal Trade Commission is charged with keeping competition both free and fair. In doing this it attempts to safeguard the public by preventing false or misleading advertising of food, drugs, cosmetics, and therapeutic devices, and by preventing deceptive practices in interstate commerce. Recent activities of this agency have included the restricting of misleading advertising associated with vitamin and food supplement plans, and restrictions against books advertising cures for a wide variety of ills.[8]

*The Post Office Department.* Existing laws permit the Post Office Department to take action against quacks who use the mails in an attempt to bilk the public in a "false or fraudulent" manner. Mail-order panaceas for obesity, arthritis, and others have recently been investigated, and their promoters prosecuted.[9] Any consumer who believes that he has discovered a fraudulent business should not hesitate to report it.

### Professional Organizations

The varied and widespread problems of consumer health are also of concern to a number of professional organizations. The American Medical Association, the American Dental Association, and the Better Business Bureau are several of these groups that are interested in helping their own members and the consumer become better informed about the products and services that they use.

---

[7] *United States Government Organization Manual 1964-65* (Washington: Government Printing Office, 1964), pp. 362-64.

[8] *Ibid.*, p. 413.

[9] Sidney W. Bishop, "Report from the Post Office Department," *Proceedings, Second National Congress on Medical Quackery,* October 25-26, 1963 (Chicago: American Medical Association, n.d.), p. 17.

The *American Medical Association's* Department of Investigation has the largest file in existence on medical quackery, and cooperates with law enforcement agencies by providing evidence leading to convictions. Because of this phase of its work, the Association has been sued numerous times in past years, but it has lost just one suit and *one cent* in damages! Other departments and committees of the Association are similarly engaged in trying to provide for the better health of the American people. Publications of the *American Dental Association* include materials on the care of the teeth, fluoridation, diet and dental health, and various pamphlets for parents and teachers. An extensive film collection, available on a rental basis, also aids in educating the school child and the citizen about the benefits of adequate and reliable dental care. The *Better Business Bureau* keeps its members (business and professional firms and their employees) informed about questionable business practices in the community by means of special bulletins, and investigates and acts upon complaints of unfair and unethical business practices. The Bureau provides a valuable public service through its many activities against unscrupulous advertising, misleading promotion schemes, and the distribution of fraudulent and worthless "cures."

### The Consumer's Choice

Being alert to the possibility of fraud and deception in the area of health products and services is one of the best ways to avoid being deceived. You can protect your health *and* your pocketbook if you will give consideration to the following recommendations when spending your dollars:

1. Rely on the advice of your physician when considering the purchase of specific products that claim health benefits.
2. Avoid the purchasing of special health foods, food supplements, and vitamins, unless they are prescribed by your physician. A well balanced diet will take care of your nutritional needs.

3. Learn to recognize the various "pitches" of the modern medicine man.
4. Be suspicious of health products sold by door-to-door salesmen.
5. Be wary of all products and mechanical devices that are claimed to be useful for the cure of arthritis, rheumatism, cancer, and other chronic diseases.
6. Be alert when reading advertisements for health products.
7. Look for proprietary drug products (nonprescription drugs) that bear the letters U.S.P. or N.F., meaning that they meet the standards of identity, purity, and strength established by the United States Pharmacopeia or National Formulary.
8. Read the labels on the products you purchase. The Food, Drug and Cosmetic Act requires that the label tell contents, what the product will do, how to use the product, and any cautions that should be observed in its use.
9. Do not hesitate to contact the Better Business Bureau, local Medical Society, Food and Drug Administration offices, or the Post Office Department if you believe you have discovered a fraudulent product or scheme.

### SELECTING YOUR HEALTH ADVISORS

Health personnel play an important role in helping you maintain positive health and in helping you return to that level following illness. The selection of competent health advisors is one of your most important duties. As a college student you probably have not been faced with this problem. At home, your family physician was selected by your parents. While you are attending college, health services may be provided by the college or university health service or by community physicians and other personnel recommended by the health service. But there will soon come a time when it will be important to understand how to select health advisors.

The term "doctor" is a confusing one. Those who legally use it before their names may be teachers, ministers, veterinarians, dentists, medical doctors, osteopathic physicians, or chiropractors. They may also be quack practitioners or self-designated "doctors"—persons who claim to have medical knowledge and skills but who are not actually qualified in this way. How can you decide which "doctor" to visit when you are in need of health care or advice? Who are the different "doctors" in the health field? What training have they had? What theories of health and disease do they believe?

### Physicians

*Medical Doctor (M.D.).* The competent and well trained physician of today is an advisor upon whom you can depend in health or illness. He provides preventive medicine services such as immunizations and health examinations, and when illness does occur, he can use drugs, surgery, and other scientific techniques to restore health. In all of his work the physician makes use of scientific research findings relative to the prevention and cure of disease.

Medical schools are highly selective in admitting students To qualify, a young man or woman must have a college academic background of high quality (including a college degree, in the vast majority of instances) and traits of personality and character that will qualify him for this field of study. Intensity of purpose is one important characteristic, for medical education consists of a rigorous four-year course of study and a minimum of one year of internship before starting to practice. If the physician decides to specialize, from two to five additional years are required after receiving the M.D. degree, and even then the physician's education is not complete. New diseases, drugs, and scientific developments are so extensive that the modern physician constantly needs to read, study, and attend institutes and seminars to keep up-to-date.

The general medical practitioner, whose practice is not limited to any one field of medical endeavor, and who may be your family physician, can call upon the services of a number of different specialists when the need arises. Some of the more common medical specialists (M.D.) are the following:

*Dermatologist*—Specializes in diagnosis and treatment of diseases of the skin and skin manifestations of constitutional diseases.

*Gynecologist*—Specializes in diseases of the female reproductive organs.

*Internist*—Specializes in diagnosis and nonsurgical treatment of diseases of the internal organs.

*Obstetrician*—Specializes in care for women during pregnancy and childbirth, and the period immediately following.

*Ophthalmologist (Oculist)*—Specializes in diagnosis and treatment of diseases and disorders of the eye and vision, and prescribes glasses.

*Orthopedist (Orthopedic Surgeon)*—Specializes in diagnosis and treatment of diseases, fractures, and deformities of the bones and joints by physical, medical, and surgical methods.

*Pediatrician*—Specializes in prevention, diagnosis, and treatment of diseases of children usually up to the age of sixteen.[10]

Some of the other medical specialties are anesthesiology, endocrinology, geriatrics, proctology, radiology, cardiology, urology, psychiatry, and surgery.

*Doctor of Osteopathy (D.O.).* Doctors of osteopathy are trained in all branches of medicine, including the use of drugs, surgery, and x-ray. In addition, the osteopathic physician is trained in manipulation. "Osteopathy contends that early symptoms of functional disease may be projected in the musculo-skeletal system of the patient. The osteopathic physician . . . often discovers these irregularities and can apply corrective treatment.[11]

---

[10] School Health Education Study, Experimental Curriculum Materials Project, "Medical Specialists" (Washington: School Health Education Study, November, 1964), pp. 1-2.

[11] American Osteopathic Association, *The Osteopathic Profession* (Chicago: The Association, n.d.).

The majority of the students in osteopathic medical schools have already received college degrees, and must show academic ability and other professional qualifications in order to be admitted. Following a four-year course of study consisting of basic sciences and clinical experiences, the osteopathic physician serves a year's internship in an approved osteopathic hospital. The osteopathic physician also may choose to specialize in obstetrics, pediatrics, pathology, and many other fields.[12]

The osteopathic physician is licensed to practice in all states and has been granted unlimited practice rights in thirty-eight states and the District of Columbia. Some states restrict the use of drugs and/or surgery by this physician.[13]

### Dentists

The dental field is considerably less complicated than the medical one. Dentists have either a *Doctor of Dental Surgery* degree *(D.D.S.)* or a *Doctor of Dental Medicine* degree *(D.M.D.)*, depending upon the degree awarded by the dental school from which they graduated. In either case, they are well trained to treat tooth, jaw, and gum diseases, and to offer preventive services such as topical fluoride applications and cleanings. Before beginning his professional training the dental student has had a minimum of three years of college (usually four) and has had to demonstrate ability and aptitude for this profession. One of the most common dental specialties is *orthodontia*, the prevention and correction of tooth irregularities.

### Additional Eye Health Personnel

We have already mentioned the *ophthalmologist (oculist)*, the medical specialist who treats diseases and disorders of the eyes and vision. There are also other personnel in this field:[14]

---

[12] *Ibid.*

[13] American Osteopathic Association, *Focus on Osteopathic Education* (Chicago: The Association, n.d.), p. 5.

[14] Mary K. Beyrer, "Medical and Dental Specialists Plus Other Health Personnel" (The Ohio State University, 1962), p. 4 (Mimeographed).

*Optometrist (O.D.)*—one whose education, training, and licensure qualify him to examine eyes, without the use of drugs, for abnormal visual problems not due to disease. He may prescribe, fit, and supply eyeglasses and provide visual training for such conditions.

*Optician*—a skilled technician who is qualified to grind lenses, fit, and dispense eyeglasses.

*Orthoptist*—trained to correct strabismus and strengthen weakened eye muscles by means of exercises prescribed by an ophthalmologist.

## Limited Practitioners

*Doctor of Chiropractic (D.C.).* Chiropractors consider their system a natural, drugless healing method, in which health is maintained by establishing a perfect alignment of the body's bone and nerve structure. They believe that all the systems and functions of the body are controlled by the nervous system, and that interference with the nerve control of these systems impairs their functioning and causes disease by making the body more susceptible to infection.[15]

High school graduation is the minimum requirement for admission to the chiropractic colleges, although approximately half the states require at least two years of pre-chiropractic college work for licensure. The college course of study is a four-year program.

*Doctor of Podiatry (Pod.D.).* The podiatrist or chiropodist *(Doctor of Surgical Chiropody, D.S.C.)* is trained to diagnose and treat a variety of foot ailments, including corns, calluses, warts, tumors, ulcers, and rashes. This doctor has received his training at a four-year college of chiropody, following at least one year of college premedical work. Although he does not treat them, he is trained to recognize symptoms of heart disease, arthritis, diabetes, and other diseases that might affect foot health, and he refers patients with these conditions to a physician.[16]

---

[15] National Chiropractic Association, *Chiropractic . . . A Career* (Webster City, Iowa: The Association, n.d.), p. 5.

[16] Ohio Chiropodists Association, *What Everyone Should Know About Foot Doctors* (Columbus: The Association, 1960).

### Other Practitioners

The consumer will occasionally become aware of several other practitioners in the health field. Mechanotherapists, naturopaths, electrotherapists, and others use different types of treatment such as sun, electricity, mechanical devices, and water in the treatment of disease. Educational requirements and professional training in these fields are varied, but are not on a level with those in the medical field. The consumer needs to be aware of the possibility of quackery in these areas.

### How to Spot a Health Quack

Certain signals should arouse your suspicions that a medical quack is looking at your pocketbook. The Department of Investigation of the American Medical Association says to beware if:[17]

1. He uses a special or "secret" formula or machine that he claims can cure diseases.
2. He promises a quick or easy cure.
3. He advertises, using "case histories" or testimonials to impress people.
4. He clamors constantly for medical investigation and recognition.
5. He claims medical men are persecuting him or that they are afraid of his competition.
6. He tells you that his method of treatment is better than surgery, x-rays, or drugs.

### How to Choose Your Health Advisors

Let us suppose, now, that you have made a decision. You know what type of medical or dental care you wish to have, but you don't know how to find it. This may seem like a simple problem, but it takes consideration and is worthy of

---

[17] American Medical Association, *Mechanical Quackery* (Chicago: The Association, 1964), p. 7.

time and effort *before* the emergency or other situation that requires medical or dental care. The following suggestions might be of assistance:

1. Ask your hometown health advisors if they can recommend advisors in your new community.
2. Ask educated, alert persons who have lived in your new community long enough to have selected health advisors. Your minister or employer might be able to make suggestions.
3. Ask the local medical and dental societies for the names of several advisors whom they would recommend in your area of the community.
4. Compare the lists of names you have. Are any advisors mentioned by several sources? This may be a sign worth noting.
5. Make an appointment to visit one or more of the physicians and dentists. Find out where they received their education, what hospital staffs they are on, whether they make home and night calls, and whether they are individuals whom you like and who appear to be sincere and professional.

If you want to learn more about the doctors on your list consult the American Medical Directory, which is available at public libraries, medical associations, and hospitals. The Directory tells the educational background, experience, professional affiliations, and special fields of interest of the physicians.

Choose your health advisors carefully. These are among the most important decisions you will ever make.

## PAYING THE COST OF HEALTH CARE

Getting your money's worth and protecting your health are similarly important in the area of health insurance. This is another consideration for you, the college student. You are probably one of the 75 per cent of the population that has some form of *health insurance*, and it is likely that you are "covered" by virtue of your parents' policy. Many policies provide for the coverage of dependent children until age nineteen or twenty. (This age varies with different insurance companies.) If you are not covered by your parents' policy, you may have a policy in your own name, available through the college or university, but sold by a private insurance company. Or, you may have purchased your own policy directly from a private firm. Married students, who need to consider protection for wives and families, ordinarily have to carry the latter type of insurance policy in order to receive the broad protection they need. Regardless of the source of one's insurance, however, it is helpful to understand what type of protection is available in different types of policies.

Perhaps we should discuss another question before going any further: Why should you have health insurance? College students are, in general, a healthy group—so why spend the money? There are no absolute answers to this question. It is true that the majority of the population will not be hospitalized or injured in any one year, but each individual needs to look at his own situation when making this decision.

Hospital care is expensive. It is not uncommon for basic expenses to be twenty-five to thirty-five dollars per day, not including special medications, extra nursing care, x-ray services, doctors' bills, and any number of additional costs that accumulate when one is ill. What reserves do you have to meet these expenses? Will you be able to draw upon your own savings or your family's? What hardships will this involve? How likely are you to become ill? Children and young adults have a high accident rate. Older people are more likely to experience illnesses. Families with young children frequently have unexpected medical expenses. These are a few of the considerations involved when you survey your need for health insurance. Most of us feel that we would rather have insurance protection, even if we do not use it.

Before purchasing insurance it is necessary to decide the type of health expenses you want to be protected against and the extent of the protection you desire. There are five different categories or types of protection available.

*Hospital insurance* provides assistance in the payment of hospital room and board charges, usual nursing care, drugs, laboratory expenses, and others. Some hospital plans provide for complete payment of all bills (with perhaps some exceptions, such as diagnostic tests or blood plasma), while others allow up to specified amounts for certain services, and the patient pays the difference between the allowance and the actual bill.

*Surgical insurance* provides for the payment of all or part of the doctor's fee for an operation.

*Regular medical expense insurance* provides benefits for the payment of doctor's home and office visits, laboratory work, and other expenses.

*Major medical or catastrophe insurance* is designed to assist in the payment of very heavy hospital and surgical bills—those that run into the thousands of dollars. Many of these policies are written with a deductible amount, like auto insurance, with the individual paying the first hundred dollars or five hundred dollars or whatever the deductible amount is, and the insurance company paying the remainder of the bill or 75 or 80 per cent of it.

*Loss-of-income insurance* pays the individual cash benefits weekly or monthly if he is unable to work due to illness or accident.

Many college students will find health insurance plans available to them through their colleges and universities at nominal rates. This is *group insurance,* similar to that available to employee groups in industry and business. Group policies are usually less expensive than similar insurance purchased individually, and the benefits may be more extensive.

Most wise consumers are good shoppers. They know quality. Quality is also important when health insurance is purchased, and after deciding what basic type you desire, there are a number of items that can help you to determine the quality of the plans presented by different companies. First, of course, do your business with a reputable insurance company. The major, well established firms offer reliable protection. Talk to their agents and compare the coverage provided by the different companies. How many hospital days are provided for? How does the allowance for hospital room and board charges compare with the hospital rates in your area? Are drugs, x-rays, special nursing services, and other expensive extra costs provided for? If you are married, are your dependents covered as fully as you are? Are maternity benefits provided? Does the "deductible" apply to each family member or to the whole family? In general, try to compare the plans, item by item, and determine which one gives you the most protection of the type you desire for the money involved. As in the purchase of other consumer goods, you generally get what you pay for.

The way in which we choose and pay for our medical services is a matter of importance to most Americans. The traditional approach, on a private physician-patient basis, is usually preferred because of the personal freedom involved and the high quality of the care received. Other types of medical care programs have developed in some areas of the country. Physicians, specialists, technicians, and others are employed by an organization and offer medical care on a teamwork basis. The Kaiser Foundation Health Plan, available in several west coast areas, and New York City's Health Insurance Plan are two well-known examples. For an annual or monthly fee, subscribers receive comprehensive medical care. You may be familiar with the Mayo Clinic in Rochester, Minnesota, or the Lahey Clinic in Boston. These are examples of clinics that also offer medical care on a teamwork basis, but payment is made according to the services rendered, as is done with one's family physician.

The progress and standards of American medicine and health care are the envy of much of the rest of the world. It is true that hospital costs seem extremely high. A day of care in the hospital has increased 278 per cent in cost in the past fifteen years and this increase has been criticized by the public. A large portion of the increase is due to steadily rising wage levels for highly trained technicians and other types of hospital employees. In addition, advances in medical science are factors in the rising costs. New drugs, surgical techniques, and diagnostic procedures all cause expenses to rise.[18] They also provide better care than has ever been available before. About 6 per cent of the average family's income is spent for health and medical services. Research data indicate that in a recent year the average person spent $129 for such services. Figure 6 indicates the way in which the consumer's health dollar is spent. Would any one of us wish to return to the medical era of the 1940's?

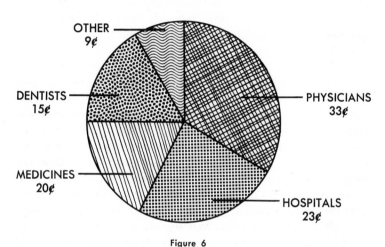

Figure 6

*How the Health Dollar Is Spent**

* National Center for Health Statistics, Vital and Health Statistics, Series 10, No. 9, Data from the National Health Survey, *Medical Care, Health Status, and Family Income,* May, 1964, pp. 47-51.

As more and more people are joining the ranks of the elderly, health care for senior citizens becomes one of the medical concerns of our country. *Medicare,* a government

---

[18] George W. Bugbee, "Planning Continued Expenditures," *Progress in Health Services* (Chicago: Health Information Foundation, May-June, 1963), p. 5.

sponsored plan, includes some medical benefits for the person over 65 in the Social Security program. Major benefits are in the areas of hospital and nursing home care; physicians' fees, most drugs, dental care, and a number of other expenses are not included. Benefits are available to everyone over 65 who is covered by Social Security, regardless of financial need.

The provision of medical care is administered in different ways in different countries. Some medical care programs for the total population are completely administered and supported by the government. In any consideration of medical care, most Americans wish the freedom to choose their own physicians and to be assured of the continued availability of high quality medical care.

## YOU ARE THE CONSUMER . . . WHAT CAN YOU DO?

There are few college students or their professors who have money to throw away, yet that is what they and many other Americans are doing daily, as they spend money and risk their lives by using worthless products and fraudulent medical care. The total bill is at least a billion dollars a year, a sum that well might be put to better use. The human cost cannot be estimated.

What factors are involved in this unnecessary waste of lives and money? *Ignorance* is undoubtedly involved in some instances. Many people do not know how to avoid a quack practitioner, do not know that at the present time diabetes can be controlled but not cured, do not know that all cancer *isn't* hopeless if it receives proper and early medical care. The college student who continues to keep up with health and medical developments should be able to protect himself from fraudulent schemes. *Today's Health,* the American Medical Association's publication for the layman, can be extremely helpful in keeping the average citizen alert and informed in the health field.

Equally as dangerous as ignorance is *apathy*, a second factor that retards health progress. The college students who use tranquilizers and/or amphetamine ("keep awake") pills; the person who knows the dangers of self-medication, but continues to use lozenges, cough medicines, and other products to treat his illnesses; these are the apathetic members of our population—the ones with the "So what?" or "Who cares?" attitude.

*Fear* is one of the greatest problems in this area of frauds and quackery. Fear of doctors and hospitals, surgery, medical examinations, and other procedures may lead persons to use products and services that assure them of cures without surgery, hospitalization, or any of the *truly* miraculous procedures that can bring better health and better living to those who avail themselves of them at an early stage of their illnesses.

If you have a broad background of information and understanding in the health field and know where to seek reliable information, you are in a position to be able to avoid the frauds and quackery that appear on the American scene. Knowledge will decrease any normal fears you may have and help you make judgments based on scientific information, rather than on the basis of hearsay, advertising, or the clever patter of a talented but misleading salesman.

For better living and positive health, consider these designs for action:

Evaluate advertisements carefully . . .

Choose health advisors in relation to their scientific training and philosophies . . .

Report suspected frauds to appropriate authorities . . .

Let your local, state, and national representatives know that you want them to support legislation designed to combat frauds . . .

BE AN INTELLIGENT CONSUMER! ! !

## Problems for Your Consideration

1. What is the responsibility of the consumer in protecting *himself* from health frauds and quackery?
2. What persons, organizations, and other resources can we consult in trying to determine the reliability of health products and services?
3. What guidelines help you make suitable choices of proprietary drug products?
4. What are the factors to consider when choosing medical and health personnel to serve you and your family?
5. What provisions are included in the health insurance policy that your family carries? Are *you* covered by this policy? Until what age?
6. What are the features of the different programs available to help solve the medical care problems of the elderly?

## Suggested References

Consumer Reports, *The Medicine Show*. Revised edition. New York: Simon and Schuster, 1963.
Deutsch, Ronald M., *The Nuts Among the Berries*. New York: Ballantine Books, Inc., 1961.
Holbrook, Stewart H., *The Golden Age of Quackery*. New York: Collier Books, 1962.
Margolius, Sidney, *A Consumer's Guide to Health Insurance Plans*. New York: Public Affairs Committee, Inc., 1962.
Smith, Ralph Lee, *The Health Hucksters*. New York: Thomas Y. Crowell Company, 1960.
———, "The Strange World of Mechanical Quackery," *Today's Health*. 42 (November, 1964), pp. 42-47, 73 f.

# GLOSSARY

**abortion** (ah-bor'shun): the premature expulsion of the embryo or fetus from the uterus; may be either spontaneous or induced.

**adjustment** (ad-just'ment): success in meeting demands and needs in a situation or/and a constantly changing environment.

**allergen** (al'er-jen): a substance which is capable of producing an allergy.

**allergy** (al'er-je): hypersensitive state acquired through exposure to a particular allergen.

**amenorrhea** (ah-men"o-rē'ah): absence or cessation of menstruation after it once has been established.

**amnion** (am"nē-on): the thin, fluid-filled, membranous sac within which the product of conception develops.

**amphetamine** (am-fet'ah-min): a type of stimulating addicting drug used in the manufacture of "pep" pills.

**anoxia** (an-ok'se-ah): a condition in which there is a lack of oxygen in the body tissues.

**antibiotic** (an"te-bī-ot'ik): a chemical product which has the capacity to inhibit the growth of or destroy bacteria. Used largely in the treatment of infectious diseases.

**antibody** (an'te-bod"e): a chemical protective substance formed by the body in response to an antigen or other foreign material.

**antigen** (an'te-jen): a substance that stimulates the production of antibodies.

**antiserum** (an"te-se'rum): a serum containing antibodies injected into individuals lacking sufficient antibodies.

**antitoxin** (an"te-tok'sin): a substance which contains antibodies to a specific toxin.

**arteriosclerosis** (ar-te"re-ō-skle-rō'sis): the condition marked by loss of elasticity, thickening and the hardening of the arterial walls.

148 Glossary

**atherosclerosis** (ath"er-ō"skle-rō'sis): a specific type of arteriosclerosis in which the hardening is produced in the inner wall of
the artery.

**basal metabolism** (ba'sal me-tab'o-lizm): the amount of energy
required to support the body when at complete rest.
**BCG (Bacillus of Calmette and Guérin):** a vaccine providing
protection against tuberculosis.
**benign** (be-nīn): nonmalignant; not recurrent.
**breech birth** (brēch berth): birth in which the buttocks or the
legs of the fetus are presented before the head.

**calorie** (kal'ō-rē): the amount of heat required to raise one gram
of water one degree centigrade. A large calorie is the amount
of heat required to raise one kilogram of water one degree
centigrade. The large calorie or kilocalorie is used in the
study of metabolism to measure the amount of energy
supplied by food to the body.
**carcinogen** (kar'si-nō-jen): any cancer-producing substance.
**carcinoma** (kar"si-nō'mah): a malignant tumor made up of epithelial
cells tending to infiltrate the surrounding tissues.
**cardiology** (kar-dē-ol'o-jē): the study of the heart and its functions.
**cardiovascular** (kar"dē-o-vas'ku-lar): pertaining to the heart and
blood vessels.
**cervix** (ser'viks): the lower, narrow end of the uterus which con-
nects with the vagina.
**cesarean section** (se-sa'rē-an): delivery of the child by an incision
through the abdominal and uterine wall.
**chancre** (shāng'ker): a pimple-like sore characterizing the primary
stage of syphilis and developing at the site of entrance of the
syphilitic infection.
**cholesterol** (ko-les'ter-ol): a fatlike, pearly substance found in
animal fats and oils; normally found in the blood and other
tissues.
**chromosome** (krō'mō-sōm): the cellular element containing the
genes which are the carriers of hereditary characteristics.
**chronic** (kron'ik): of long duration, not acute.
**clitoris** (kli'to-ris): a small body of erectile tissue, situated at the
anterior angle of the vulva.
**coitus** (ko'i-tus): sexual intercourse.
**colitis** (ko-li'tis): inflammation of the colon.

collateral circulation (ko-lat'er-al): the establishment of an alternate blood supply when the primary supply has been partially or totally occluded.

communicable disease (ko-mu'ni-kah-b'l): a condition which is capable of being transmitted from one person to another.

conception (kon-sep'shun): the act of penetration of an ovum by a sperm.

congenital (kon-jen'i-tal): existing at, and usually before, birth.

contraception (kon"trah-sep'shun): the prevention of conception or impregnation.

coronary thrombosis (kor'ō-na-rē throm-bō'sis): "heart attack," formation of a blood clot in one of the arteries supplying blood to the heart.

dental caries (ka're-ēs): tooth decay; a disease of the calcified parts of the teeth resulting from the action of microorganisms on carbohydrates.

depressant (de-pres'ant): a substance which reduces functional activity by producing muscular relaxation.

DNA (Desoxyribonucleic acid) (des-ok"sē-re"bō-nu'kle-ik): a tightly coiled, double-spiral structure which transmits hereditary information, controls protein manufacture, and administrates all body structure and function.

dysmenorrhea (dis"men-ō-re'ah): painful menstruation.

ejaculation (ē-jak"u-la'shun): a sudden act of expulsion, as of the semen during sexual excitement.

embryo (em'bre-ō): the developing individual from one week after conception to the end of the third month.

emphysema (em"fi-sē'mah): a condition in which exhalation of air from the lungs is made difficult due to obstruction and loss of the lungs' elasticity; shortness of breath results.

endocarditis (en"dō-kar-dī'tis): inflammation of the endocardium, the lining of the heart, the endocardium.

endocrinologist (en"dō-kri-nol'ō-jist): a physician who treats diseases arising from disordered endocrine glands.

epididymis (ep"i-did'i-mis): a long, coiled tube which collects and stores sperm; attached to the upper part of each testicle.

erection (e-rek'shun): the condition of being made rigid and elevated due to sexual excitement.

**erythroblastosis fetalis** (e-rith"rō-blast-tō'sis fe-ta'lis): anemic condition in fetal life or soon after birth due to Rh incompatibility between the blood of the mother and the fetus.

**estrogen** (es'tro-jen): female sex hormone.

**etiolcgy** (e"te-ol'o-je): the study or theory of the cause of any disease.

**fallopian tube** (fah-lō'pe-an): a tube which conveys the ova from an ovary to the uterus.

**fertilization** (fer'ti-lī-zā'shun): the fusion of the sperm with an ovum.

**fetus** (fē'tus): the designation for the developing young in the human uterus from the end of the third month until its birth.

**fluoridation** (floo-or"i-da'shun): the addition of fluoride to the public water as part of the public health program to prevent or reduce the incidence of dental caries.

**fraternal twins:** two offspring produced in the same pregnancy and developed from two ova fertilized at the same time by two sperm; coincidental pregnancies.

**genes** (jēns): the units of which chromosomes are composed; the carriers of hereditary characteristics.

**genetics** (je-net'iks): the study of heredity.

**genital organs** (jen'i-tal): the reproductive organs.

**geriatrics** (jer"ē-at'riks): the branch of medicine which treats all problems and diseases of old age and aging.

**gestation** (jes-tā'shun): the period of pregnancy, the condition of having a developing embryo or fetus in the body.

**heterosexual** (het"er-ō-seks'u-al): pertaining to the opposite sex.

**heterozygous** (het"er-ō-zī'gus): inheritance of both dominant and recessive genes from parents to form one particular, physical characteristic.

**homosexual** (hō"mō-seks'u-al): pertaining to the same sex.

**hormone** (hor'mōn): a chemical substance secreted by an endocrine gland and carried to other parts of the body where it affects the activities of other organs.

**hymen** (hī'men): the membranous fold which partially or wholly covers the external opening of the vagina.

**hypertension** (hī"per-ten'shun): abnormally high blood pressure.

**identical twins:** two offspring of the same sex developed from one fertilized ovum which divides.

**immunity** (i-mu'ni-tē): a high degree of resistance to specific organisms; dependent upon antibodies.

**infectious agent** (in-fek'shus): an organism capable of producing infection.

**infertility** (in"fer-til'i-te): an inability to reproduce young because of inherited or acquired defects; sometimes correctable.

**insulin** (in'su-lin): a hormone formed by the islands of Langerhans in the pancreas and secreted into the blood where it regulates carbohydrate (sugar) metabolism; used in treating diabetes.

**labor** (lā'bor): the means by which the fetus is expelled from the uterus through the vagina to the outside world.

**lactation** (lak-tā'shun): the secretion of milk.

**lesion** (lē'zhun): any local abnormality or change in body tissue: bruise, wound, inflammation, tumor, cavity, etc.

**leukemia** (lu-kē'mē-ah): a disease of the blood-forming organs, characterized by a marked increase in the number of white blood cells.

**malignant** (mah-lig'nant): a tumor that has the ability to metastasize; commonly used in referring to cancer.

**masturbation** (mas"tur-bā'shun): self-stimulation of one's sex organs.

**menarche** (me-nar'kē): the establishment or beginning of the menstrual function.

**menopause** (men'-o-pawz): cessation of menstruation in the human female, occurring usually between the age of 46 and 50.

**menstruation** (men-stroo-a'shun): the monthly discharge of uterine lining which occurs when the ovum has not been fertilized.

**metastasis** (me-tas'tah-sis): the transfer of disease from one organ or part of an organ to another area of the body not directly connected to the diseased portion.

**miscarriage** (mis-car'age): premature birth or expulsion of an embryo or fetus before it is able to maintain life; spontaneous abortion.

**morbidity** (mor-bid'i-tē): the presence of disease; also the ratio of sick to well persons in a community.

**mortality** (mor-tal'i-tē): death; also the death rate; the ratio of total number of deaths to the total population.

**neurosis** (nū-rō'sis): a mild mental disorder which hinders effective daily living.

**N.F. (National Formulary):** drugs marked with N.F. have met the standards of identity, purity, and strength established by a committee of the American Pharmaceutical Association.

**nocturnal emissions** (nok-tur'nal e-mish'un): "wet dream;" reflex discharge of the semen during sleep.

**nostrum** (nos'trum): a quack, patent, or secret remedy.

**noncommunicable disease:** a condition which is not capable of being transmitted from one person to the other.

**obesity** (o-bes'i-te): excessive overweight; an increase in body weight beyond the limitation of skeletal and physical requirement.

**orgasm** (or'gazm): the climax of intense sexual excitement.

**ovary** (ō'vah-rē): the female sexual gland in which the ova are produced.

**ovulation** (ōv"u-lā'shun): the discharge of a mature, unimpregnated ovum from the follicle of the ovary.

**ovum** (ō'vum): egg; female reproductive cell which, after fertilization, develops into a new member of the same species.

**"Pap" (Papanicolaou's test)** (Pap"ah-nik"o-la'ōōz): a method of staining smears of various body secretions, for example, those shed by the uterine lining; used to detect the presence of a malignant process.

**pathogen** (path'ō-jen): any organism, or agent, capable of producing disease.

**penis** (pē'nis): male sex organ.

**personality** (per"su-nal'i-tē): that which constitutes, distinguishes, and characterizes a person; the total reaction of a person to his environment.

**phenylketonuria (PKU)** (fen"il-ke"to-nu're-ah): an hereditary defect in an enzyme of the liver due to paired recessive genes; results in an inability to metabolize the protein phenylalanine. This condition is associated with mental defects.

**placenta** (plah-sen'tah): vascular mass within the uterus through which the fetus is nourished by means of the umbilical cord.

**premature birth** (pre-mah-tūr'): occurring before the normal gestation period has been completed.

**premature infant** (pre-mah-tūr): one with a birth weight of less than five-and-one-half pounds.

**proctology** (prok-tol'o-je): the branch of medicine treating the rectum and its diseases.

**proprietary drug** (pro-prī'e-ta-rē): nonprescription drugs; for reliability and safety look for those that bear the letters U.S.P. or N.F., and read directions on labels.

**prostate gland** (pros'tāt): a gland surrounding the neck of the bladder and the urethra in the male.

**psychiatry** (sī-kī'ah-trē): that branch of medicine which deals with mental and emotional disorders.

**psychosis** (sī-kō'sis): a mental illness characterized by a loss of contact with reality; a departure from normal standards of thinking, feeling, and acting.

**psychosomatic** (sī"kō-so-mat'ik): pertaining to the mind-body relationship; having bodily symptoms of a psychic, emotional, or mental origin.

**puberty** (pū'ber-tē): the age at which the reproductive organs become functionally operative and secondary sex characteristics develop.

**quack** (kwak): one who makes fake medical claims having no widely accepted authoritative basis.

**RAD or Radiation Absorbed Dose:** refers to the measure of energy imparted to matter by ionizing particles per unit mass of the irradiated material.

**radiation** (rā"dē-ā'shun): the giving off of rays; also the rays themselves, as heat rays, light rays, x-rays; one of the accepted treatments for cancer.

**radioisotope** (rā"de-ō-ī'sō-tōp): radioactive elements used for both diagnosis and treatment; can be used as tracers or as destroyers of diseased tissue.

**radiology** (rā"dē-ol'ō-jē): the branch of medicine which deals with the use of radiant energy in the diagnosis and treatment of disease.

**resistance** (re-zis'tans): the ability of the tissues to withstand or ward off infection.

**Rh factor:** an inherited blood characteristic of no concern unless an Rh-negative woman marries an Rh-positive man and conceives an Rh-positive baby. In this case, infant may develop erythroblastosis fetalis.

**roentgen** (rent'gen): the international unit of radiation used as x-rays for diagnostic and therapeutic medicine.

**rubella** (roo-bel'ah): German measles: fever with a rash characteristically lasting about three days. When it occurs during the first three months of pregnancy, it may produce severe fatal malformations.

**rubeola** (roo-bē'ō-lah): old-fashioned measles: characterized by a fever followed by a diffuse red rash; lasts approximately two weeks.

**saturated fat:** category of foods of animal origin; considered high in cholesterol.

**schizophrenia** (skiz"ō-fre'nē-ah): a type of psychosis characterized by loss of contact with environment and by disintegration and cleavage of the personality.

**scrotum** (skrō'tum): the pouch which contains the testicles and their accessory organs.

**semen** (sē'men): the thick, whitish, sperm-containing secretion of the reproductive organs in the male.

**seminal vesicle** (sem'i-nal ves'i-cle): a sac-like gland in which semen is stored; attached to the bladder.

**spermatozoa or sperm** (sper"mah-tō-zō'ah): male reproductive cell produced in the testes.

**spirochete** (spī'rō-kēt): a spiral-shaped bacterium; one type causes syphilis.

**sterility** (ste-ril'ī-tē): inability to reproduce young.

**stroke** (strōk): cerebral vascular accident caused by a thrombus or the rupture of an artery in a portion of the brain.

**"subclinical deficiency":** a condition in which it is not possible to obtain any evidence of a deficiency; proposed by food fadists as a reason for vitamin supplements.

**subclinical deficiency:** an infection which is not severe enough to produce the typical symptoms of the disease.

**symptomatic** (simp"to-mat'ik): pertaining to the nature of a symptom; the functional evidence of a disease or of a patient's condition.

**syndrome** (sin'drōm): a set of symptoms which occur together in a characteristic manner.

**tension** (ten'shun): the condition of being under physical or mental stress.

**tertiary syphilis** (ter′shē-er-ē sif′i-lis): the third stage of syphilis characterized by cardiovascular or central nervous system involvement.

**testis** (tes′tis): one of two male reproductive glands, situated in the scrotum, which produce sperm.

**testicle** (tes′te-k′l): the testis.

**thalidomide:** a type of tranquilizer which has been proven to cause fetal malformations when taken by the mother during the first three months of pregnancy; not approved for sale in the United States.

**thrombus** (throm′bus): a clot formed by coagulation of the blood; remains at the point of its formation in a blood vessel or in one of the cavities of the heart.

**toxemia** (toks-e′me-ah): a form of blood poisoning due to the absorption of bacterial products (toxins) formed at a local source of infection.

**toxin** (tok′sin): a poison produced by living organisms, usually bacteria.

**toxoid** (tok′soid): a product formed by treating a toxin with certain physical or chemical agents thus modifying its effect on the body; used in artificial immunization.

**tranquilizer** (trang′kwil-iz″er): a type of drug used to calm the nervous, anxious, neurotic, or psychotic patient; acts on the central nervous system.

**tuberculin test** (tu-ber′ku-lin): the injection of tuberculin—a substance consisting of the bacillus which causes tuberculosis—under or into the skin; determines the presence of tubercle bacillus in the body.

**umbilical cord** (um-bil′i-kal): the connecting link between the fetus and the placenta.

**urethra** (ū-rē′thrah): a membranous canal which conveys urine from the bladder to the surface; in the male it also carries the semen.

**urology** (ū-rol′ō-jē): branch of medicine which is concerned with the genito-urinary tract.

**U.S.P. (United States Pharmacopeia):** drugs marked with U.S.P. have met the standards of identity, purity, and strength established by the U.S.P. Convention, Inc., a non-profit organization that strives to maintain the integrity of drug products.

**uterus** (ū′ter-us): the hollow, muscular organ within which the embryo and fetus develop.


**vaccine** (vak′sēn): a preparation of toxoid or dead or weakened pathogens used for immunization.

**vagina** (vah-jī′nah): the genital canal in the female extending from the vulva to the cervix; also referred to as the birth canal.

**vector** (vek′tor): a carrier; an insect or other agent which transfers an infective agent from one host to another.

**vehicle** (vē′hi-k'l): a carrier of elements; enables the indirect transfer of disease; i.e., milk, water, food, soil, insects.

**virulence** (vir′ū-lens): the disease-producing power of a microorganism.

**vitamin supplement:** special vitamin preparation needed by the average person only when prescribed by a physician.


**X and Y chromosomes:** carriers of the genes which determine sex.

# INDEX